The Journey to Excellence in Esthetic Dentistry

Editors

YAIR Y. WHITEMAN
DAVID J. WAGNER

DENTAL CLINICS OF NORTH AMERICA

www.dental.theclinics.com

October 2020 • Volume 64 • Number 4

ELSEVIER

1600 John F. Kennedy Boulevard • Suite 1800 • Philadelphia, Pennsylvania, 19103-2899

http://www.dental.theclinics.com

DENTAL CLINICS OF NORTH AMERICA Volume 64, Number 4
October 2020 ISSN 0011-8532, ISBN: 978-0-323-75558-0

Editor: John Vassallo; j.vassallo@elsevier.com
Developmental Editor: Laura Fisher

Dental Clinics of North America (ISSN 0011-8532) is published quarterly by Elsevier Inc., 360 Park Avenue South, New York, NY 10010-1710. Months of issue are January, April, July, and October. Business and Editorial Offices: 1600 John F. Kennedy Boulevard, Suite 1800, Philadelphia, PA 19103-2899. Periodicals postage paid at New York, NY and additional mailing offices. Subscription prices are $304.00 per year (domestic individuals), $633.00 per year (domestic institutions), $100.00 per year (domestic students/residents), $366.00 per year (Canadian individuals), $821.00 per year (Canadian institutions), $100.00 per year (Canadian students/residents) $424.00 per year (international individuals), $821.00 per year (international institutions), and $200.00 per year (international students/residents). International air speed delivery is included in all *Clinics* subscription prices. All prices are subject to change without notice. **POSTMASTER:** Send address changes to *Dental Clinics of North America*, Elsevier Health Sciences Division, Subscription Customer Service, 3251 Riverport Lane, Maryland Heights, MO 63043. **Customer Service (orders, claims, online, change of address): Elsevier Health Sciences Division, Subscription Customer Service, 3251 Riverport Lane, Maryland Heights, MO 63043. Tel: 1-800-654-2452 (U.S. and Canada). Fax: 314-447-8029. E-mail: journalscustomerservice-usa@elsevier.com (for print support); journalsonlinesupport-usa@elsevier. com (for online support).**

Reprints. For copies of 100 or more, of articles in this publication, please contact the Commercial Reprints Department, Elsevier Inc., 360 Park Avenue South, New York, NY 10010-1710. Tel.: 212-633-3874; Fax: 212-633-3820; E-mail: reprints@elsevier.com.

The Dental Clinics of North America is covered in *MEDLINE/PubMed (Index Medicus), Current Contents/Clinical Medicine, ISI/BIOMED* and *Clinahl*.

Contributors

EDITORS

YAIR Y. WHITEMAN, DMD
Associate Clinical Professor, Director of Advanced Restorative and Esthetic Dentistry, Division of Constitutive and Regenerative Science, UCLA School of Dentistry, Los Angeles, California, USA

DAVID J. WAGNER, DDS
Private Practice, West Hollywood, California, USA; Clinical Lecturer, Advanced Restorative and Esthetic Dentistry, Division of Constitutive and Regenerative Science, UCLA School of Dentistry, Los Angeles, California

AUTHORS

PHIL BRISEBOIS, BA
Digital Specialist, UCLA Center for Esthetic Dentistry Lecturer, Founder NOVO Dental Studios & GRAVIDEE

SIVAN FINKEL, DMD
Advanced Program for International Dentists in Esthetic Dentistry, New York University College of Dentistry, The Dental Parlour, New York, New York

LAWRENCE FUNG, DDS
UCLA Center for Esthetic Dentistry Lecturer, Culver City, California

MARC HAYASHI, DMD, MBA
Health Sciences Assistant Clinical Professor, Section of Restorative Dentistry, UCLA School of Dentistry, Los Angeles, California

JULIE LOGAN
Writing and Branding Consultant, Los Angeles, California

ALIREZA MOSHAVERINIA, DDS, MS, PhD, FACP
Assistant Professor, Diplomate, American Board of Prosthodontics, Division of Advanced Prosthodontics, UCLA School of Dentistry, Los Angeles, California

PETER PIZZI, CDT, MDT
Advanced Program for International Dentists in Esthetic Dentistry, New York University College of Dentistry, New York, New York; Pizzi Dental Studio, Staten Island, New York

KATHRYN PRESTON, DDS, MS
Assistant Clinical Professor, Section of Orthodontics, UCLA School of Dentistry, Los Angeles, California

TODD R. SCHOENBAUM, DDS, MS
Clinical Professor, UCLA, Los Angeles, California

Contributors

PHONG TRAN CAO, DDS
Lecturer, University of California, Los Angeles, Los Angeles, California; Cosmetic Dentist and Private Practice, 5 Star Dental, Las Vegas, Nevada

DAVID WAGNER, DDS
Private Practice, West Hollywood, California, USA; Clinical Lecturer, Advanced Restorative and Esthetic Dentistry, Division of Constitutive and Regenerative Science, UCLA School of Dentistry, Los Angeles, California

YAIR Y. WHITEMAN, DMD
Associate Clinical Professor, Director of Advanced Restorative and Esthetic Dentistry, Division of Constitutive and Regenerative Science, UCLA School of Dentistry, Los Angeles, California

Contents

> This article informs dental clinicians on the essential workings of scientific research and statistical analyses. It provides clinicians with the essential knowledge necessary to understand and review scientific work.

> Material selection is one of the most important decisions to be made by clinicians. Proper material selection can affect the long-term function, longevity, and esthetics of restorations. There are a large number of restorative materials available, which has increased the complexity of the decision-making process. Improper material selection can lead to failures in the outcome. This article is designed to provide the practitioner with up-to-date practical information on ceramic restorative materials and techniques in a clear, evidence-based, and unbiased manner. It also provides decision-making guides to help the practitioner determine the best ceramic material for various clinical scenarios.

> Successful adhesive dentistry begins with correct placement and polymerization of the bonding agent. Although numerous agents exist, all abide by certain key principles, including the newest group, the universal adhesives. Fundamental steps also exist in the application process that require the operator to understand the chemistry of the adhesive being used. Modalities exist that can help preserve the durability of the bond achieved, thus slowing down the degradation process. However, no material or agent can overcome poor technique. Thus, it is of the utmost importance that the practitioner respects the technique sensitivity of adhesives, and follows the manufacturer's instructions.

> The use of digital dentistry is on the increase as costs to acquire digital technology have gone down dramatically and allowed for more practitioners to integrate digital equipment with reduced investment. One of

the most significant benefits of digital technology in dentistry is the ability to streamline processes that can be cumbersome via the analog way. In digital dentistry, it is important to understand the advantages and disadvantages of each device or system available.

Physical appearance and attractiveness consciously and subconsciously, affect patients' quality of life. Traditionally, dentists were tasked with improving a patient's smile, a central aspect of facial aesthetics and physical appearance. More recently, as the scope of practice of the aesthetic dentist has broadened to potentially include other components of facial cosmesis that go hand-in-hand with a patient's smile, new options have emerged with which modern aesthetic dentists should familiarize themselves. As laws surrounding their use in dental offices continue to evolve, Botox and dermal fillers represent natural next steps in aesthetic dentistry.

Team Collaboration and Communication

Photography is one of the most important skills dentists need to master in order to perform esthetic dentistry at a high level. Today, digital single-lens reflex cameras are commonplace. Young dentists have grown up with Internet, smartphones, and online platforms exposing them, and their patients, to cases that other dentists have shared, increasing the awareness and popularity of esthetic-focused treatment. This article provides readers with a simplified and attainable approach to begin the dental photography journey, as well as increase skill level, depending on practice style and desired investment.

No matter how skilled and well trained esthetic dentists or technicians may be, they cannot deliver results without a proper partnership. Close ceramist-clinician communication is a critical component of successful esthetic dentistry. In order to design an esthetic vision, convey this vision to the patient, and then execute the vision successfully, there must be effective communication between the ceramist, the clinician, and (most importantly) the patient. This article highlights some of the authors' philosophies, as well as an overview of the key communication protocols that have proved effective for this team.

As both restorative dentists and specialists have their respective realms of expertise, it is important to develop a team of qualified providers to improve treatment outcomes for patients. In many cases, this involves collaboration between a restorative dentist and orthodontist. Effective communication is critical, with the dentist's understanding of basic orthodontic terminology and case planning considerations. Recognizing the context in which to apply normative occlusal and cephalometric values often necessitates comprehensive specialty-level experience. All providers should recognize when to involve the indicated team members when complex multidisciplinary treatment needs are present. The team approach offers an opportunity to optimize excellent patient care.

Yair Y. Whiteman

Ideally, Orthodontic-Restorative cases are planned alongside from the beginning, however, in some instances the restorative dentist encounters the patient for esthetic evaluation near the end of orthodontic phase. This is a high-stakes evaluation because the decision to remove brackets implies that refinement of tooth positioning cannot occur unless the patient re-enters orthodontic treatment. One challenge in multidisciplinary treatment is accommodating effective communication between providers and employing Digital Smile Design outline tool as a visual aid can help optimizing treatment outcome. This article discusses the importance and steps utilizing digital outline tool to provide quick and effective communication on treatment progress and recommendations.

Business Professional Focus

David J. Wagner and Julie Logan

The objective of this article is to introduce the concept of branding to dentists interested in implementing elective esthetic treatment into their practice. For many, this will serve as an introduction to begin; for others, it can provide a road map for revising and reinforcing a branding program already in place.

DENTAL CLINICS OF NORTH AMERICA

SERIES OF RELATED INTEREST

Atlas of the Oral and Maxillofacial Surgery Clinics
http://www.oralmaxsurgeryatlas.theclinics.com

Oral and Maxillofacial Surgery Clinics
http://www.oralmaxsurgery.theclinics.com

THE CLINICS ARE AVAILABLE ONLINE!
Access your subscription at:
www.theclinics.com

Preface

The Journey to Excellence in Esthetic Dentistry

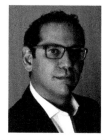 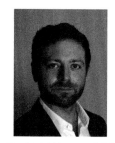

Yair Y. Whiteman, DMD   David J. Wagner, DDS
Editors

Our ability to provide patients with the most up-to-date treatment options, materials, treatment modalities, and evidence-based decision making requires a culture of continuous learning, collaborative teamwork, and exceptional focus. In his influential work, *Outliers,* Malcolm Gladwell claims that an average of 10,000 hours is required for a person to become an expert in a certain field. In dentistry, a considerable amount of time outside of "normal work hours" is necessary in order to develop skills to become an expert. This is not only where dentistry becomes a vocation, but also how we can differentiate ourselves and how we can reach and maintain satisfying and fulfilling careers.

Though dental school strives to provide students with as much in-depth knowledge and experience as possible, due to lack of time, only a foundational level of education can be achieved. As a result of continuous advancements in material science, techniques, dental research, and integration of digital technology, there has been a tremendous increase in teaching requirements and need for curriculum transformation in recent years. Consequently, dental schools may only have the bandwidth to concentrate on procedural-teaching and single-tooth dentistry. Therefore, upon graduation, when a dentist aims to practice at the highest level, they must continuously elevate their skills not only to match the latest standards of care but also to improve their ability to provide exceptional dental care beyond what is normally expected.

In this series of articles, we focus on a journey to excellence in esthetic restorative dentistry and aim to provide a roadmap for clinicians who wish to develop clinical skills and elevate the scope and status of their dental practices. We emphasize not only that at the core of this area of dental care is one's ability to technically perform treatment but also it is equally as important to attract patients, build relationships, and communicate the value of treatment. Finally, the series of articles is designed to include

Dent Clin N Am 64 (2020) ix–xi
https://doi.org/10.1016/j.cden.2020.07.004
0011-8532/20/© 2020 Published by Elsevier Inc.

dental.theclinics.com

checklists and practical reference guides that can be used while working clinically or when developing the business and team of one's practice.

To achieve a higher level of competence, dentists must pursue continuing education that is taught by ethically responsible experts rooted in sound, unbiased information. Dentists should seek out upper-echelon dental academy meetings and surround themselves with like-minded people, building lasting professional relationships with mentorship dynamics. Evidence-based scientific data must be critically evaluated and assessed when making decisions. To start, Dr Todd R. Schoenbaum provides a detailed guide for reading and evaluating scientific literature.

Materials and bonding techniques must be thoroughly understood in order to execute a minimally invasive modern style of dentistry. An update of current materials and bonding techniques is reviewed by Dr Alireza Moshaverinia and Dr Marc Hayashi. In today's dental landscape, digital technology is increasingly becoming a viable and alternative method to traditional analog workflows. Dr Lawrence Fung and digital lab innovator Mr Phil Brisebois discuss digital technology and its place and integration in the dental practice. Adjunctive services, such as injectables, have been a complementary component of the esthetic dental landscape for some time. There is a major position for their place within the scope of treatment, and patient's outcomes can be enhanced, creating an even greater value and awareness for the life-changing treatment that esthetic dentists can provide, as outlined by Dr Phong Tran Cao.

Team collaboration and communication are imperative to a dentist's success when performing restorative esthetic treatment. Photography is a tool used to help achieve seamless communication among the dental team as well as with patients. A beginner's guide to dental photography along with a clinical reference manual is provided by Dr David J. Wagner. It is known that dental esthetic treatment results hinge on the skill set of both restorative dentist and ceramist. Developing a world-class dentist-ceramist partnership is discussed by Dr Sivan Finkel and master ceramist Mr Peter Pizzi.

The role that specialists play is invaluable when properly executing minimally invasive esthetic treatment. The goal should always be to preserve as much natural tooth structure in order to accomplish the best outcome for the patient. An understanding of what is possible with various specialty points of view is therefore necessary for restorative dentists. Proper communication with all specialist types is imperative. Specifically, orthodontists play a significant role within the scope of minimally invasive treatment. Getting teeth in the proper position results in the need to reduce less tooth structure to obtain beautiful, lasting outcomes. The paired articles by orthodontist Dr Kathryn Preston and prosthodontist Dr Yair Y. Whiteman help to introduce these concepts and display a high-level communication style to allow seamless treatment integration among patient, restorative, and specialist.

Last, it is within the private practice sector that a dentist tends to find his or her professional life butterflied most, wearing multiple hats as a health care provider, a small business owner, a manager of people and the lead decision maker influencing the success of a dental practice enterprise. As we become clinicians choosing to elevate our practices, skills, patient experience, and ultimately help to change the lives of our patients by providing the highest level of dentistry that is possible, we need to be able to communicate to patients what this means. Branding is a mechanism that allows this communication to occur on many levels. To develop a brand for a dental practice in parallel with an elevated set of clinical skills can catapult a dental practice and patient experience to new heights and help to create a legacy of excellence in a world of average. Branding for the esthetic dentist is outlined by Dr David J. Wagner and Ms Julie Logan, a branding specialist based in Los Angeles, California.

We hope you find this series of articles helpful at whatever point you are in the journey to esthetic excellence. We too are on this lifelong journey and continue to seek advancement, always aiming to improve, acquire new skills and perspective, build professional relationships, and learn something new every day.

Yair Y. Whiteman, DMD
Division of Constitutive and
Regenerative Science
UCLA School of Dentistry
10833 Le-Conte Avenue
Room 33-064A CHS
Los Angeles, CA 90095-1668, USA

David J. Wagner, DDS
8733 Beverly Boulevard
Suite 202
West Hollywood, CA 90048, USA

E-mail addresses:
ywhiteman@dentistry.ucla.edu (Y.Y. Whiteman)
davidjohnwagner@gmail.com (D.J. Wagner)

Science in the Practice of Clinical Dentistry

Todd R. Schoenbaum, DDS, MS

KEYWORDS

• Biostatistics • Clinical dentistry • Science

KEY POINTS

- Comprehend study design and its impact on research quality and meaning.
- Learn essential biostatistical tests and analyses.
- Understand what is meant by statistical significance and its relation to clinical significance.

THE RATIONALE AND CHALLENGES OF IMPLEMENTING SCIENTIFIC DATA INTO CLINICAL PRACTICE

Extensive amounts of time and energy are spent by clinicians learning how to be the most proficient operators they can be, learning how to execute treatment at increasingly exceptional levels. They know that their skills, materials, techniques, diagnostic abilities, and treatment planning abilities ultimately determine how successful they are in addressing the needs and desires of their patients.

Clinical decision making is a complex skill. It requires the synthesis of hundreds of questions for every decision: material selection, preparation design, implant locations, and so forth. Some of these complex decisions are made out of habit or tradition, where clinicians rely (not necessarily incorrectly) on their mentors, previous successes, and training. Ultimately, clinicians must continue to evaluate and adapt and learn and move forward in producing improved results. Clinicians must strive to be perpetual students, to continually endeavor to improve their skills and knowledge. These improvements might be in longevity, aesthetics, ease of use, patient comfort, patient health, duration of treatment, economics, or consistency.

When making any clinical decision, there are 4 areas to take into consideration:

1. Patient desires (ie, finances, time constraints, aesthetics)
2. Clinical evaluation (ie, bone volume, American Society of Anesthesiologists classification, functional loads)
3. Unique clinical experience (eg, "We have been very successful immediately loading implants in our practice")

UCLA, 10833 Le Conte Avenue, CHS, Room B3-034, Los Angeles, CA 90095, USA
E-mail address: tschoenb@ucla.edu

Dent Clin N Am 64 (2020) 609–619
https://doi.org/10.1016/j.cden.2020.06.004
0011-8532/20/© 2020 Elsevier Inc. All rights reserved.

dental.theclinics.com

4. Scientific evidence (ie, most systematic reviews show little increase in risk for immediate load implant protocols when carefully selected and skillfully executed)

None of these 4 areas should be neglected, although at times clinicians may find
that the strength of one outweighs another. Their patients will be best served, and their
outcomes improved, when clinicians successfully incorporate as much information as
possible from each area. Scientific studies are not the be-all and end-all of clinical decision making. It represents only a piece. Clinicians' anecdotal experiences should
carry weight in the decision-making process. Conflicts arise between what clinicians
have seen to be true, in their hands, and the scientific literature. The potential reasons
for this may include differences in patient populations, differences in surgical
approach, differences in implant systems, and differences in the skill of technicians.
Individual clinicians develop standard operating procedures based on the unique situation but efforts should be made to increase the understanding of when alternative
materials and techniques should be implemented for a given clinical scenario. Expertise is built on accurate answers to hundreds of questions from all 4 areas in every clinical decision that clinicians make.

However, this article is about the science part of this process. The other 3 areas are
not addressed here but should in no way be neglected. Properly interpreted and understood, scientific evidence can significantly improve results. Scientific studies give
insight into the expected success rates of a new material, complications that can be
expected with a particular treatment protocol, or which patients might be at increased
risk for failures.

There are a few requirements, though: the science must be sound, the analysis
appropriate, the question answered relevant, and the interpretation cautious. The
job of clinicians is not to determine whether the science was sound or whether the statistical analysis was appropriate. That is the job of biostatisticians, editors, and re-
viewers. The job of clinicians is to determine whether the study question being
answered is relevant to the current bigger clinical question. Clinicians must also determine whether the interpretation of the study is correct. It is all too common in the scientific literature to see conclusion statements woefully undersupported or even
countered by the data in the study.

A Hypothetical Vignette

Imagine that a new 1-piece implant has come to market with US Food and Drug
Administration (FDA) approval. Clinicians are interested in switching over to it for
most of their implants and the patients are asking for it, but will it work? This is not
a binary question, and perhaps there will be indications where it will and will not prove
sufficiently successful. There is no objective threshold for success. What one clinician
might classify as successful might be intolerable to another. At any rate, clinicians are
considering surgically implanting this new device into a vast number of their patients
and results matter.

The clinicians ask a manufacturer representative to come by the office. They are
shown a bar graph from an osseointegration study published in a reputable journal,
and the new implant's bar is the tallest. It has superior bone to implant contact
compared with the control, and in another study, this one testing dry static axial
load to failure, the new implant's number is the biggest and there is a P value of
.02. Then there is a quote from a supposedly famous dentist: she loves the new
implant and so do her patients.

So far, everything looks promising and the clinicians decide to switch over to the
new implant. For 12 months, many of the implants placed in the practice are the

new implant; hundreds of them. The patients are happy, and the referrals are flowing in, but then the failures begin to show up. Slowly at first, then en masse. Peri-implantitis, prostheses repeatedly debonding, abutments fracturing. It seems that osseointegration and dry static axial load to failure are not the only factors that the clinicians should have considered before aggressively incorporating this material.

Looking back, the clinicians wonder how this implant got through the FDA clearance process. Without going into the granular details of the process, suffice to say that dental devices are generally FDA approved without need for extensive testing of safety and efficacy. In general, it is done by claiming (to the FDA) that the new device or material is largely similar to previously approved devices. So what did the clinicians miss in their cursory evaluation of this implant and what should they have done differently? Assuming the 2 studies they flipped through were properly performed and analyzed, the osseointegration and dry static axial load of the implant are as good as or superior to the current implants. However, those are only 2 of the hundreds of questions clinicians should be asking about whether or not this implant is viable. This implant is 1 piece, so why are none of the other implants clinicians use of this design? What are the clinical challenges of this design? Are the results of a dry static axial load test really correlated with how implants are treated in the oral environment? Is there a better way clinicians should test load to failure? Was the famous dentist raving about this implant vested in the manufacturer?

I am proposing that, in this scenario and hundreds of others like it, clinicians will be better able to identify and avoid potential problems if they have an understanding of the literature. Science cannot avoid all problems in clinical dentistry, but I hope that this article helps provide a start on a journey of better understanding of the scientific literature that clinicians rely on (directly or indirectly) to make clinical judgements. A proficient understanding of the science and literature will not occur immediately. It takes time and effort. As a starting point, I suggest that clinicians make a habit of finding a reputable, scientifically based, clinically oriented journal in their area of focus and read through it on a regular basis. This habit will increase familiarity and comfort with how studies are performed, analyzed, and interpreted. The learning curve may be steep at first. Ignore studies that are of no interest. Read through the others with the understanding that it is not necessary to grasp every aspect of what is presented. With time, a greater level of comfort and confidence will develop and I believe the reader will become significantly more empowered to make strong, science-backed decisions.

TYPES OF STUDIES AND THEIR VALUE IN CLINICAL PRACTICE

Most clinicians have seen something like the hierarchy of evidence pyramid (**Fig. 1**). A few things about this: it is not universally agreed on and various disciplines in medicine and dentistry have variations they lean on (more than 80 such hierarchies have been published). Epidemiology uses a vry different hierarchy than orthopedic surgery for example. Nor does the pyramid mean that any conclusion from an upper level is always more correct than a conclusion from a lower level. **Table 1** provides a brief explanation of the various types of studies and their use in clinical dentistry.

The hierarchy is not a strict ranking of what study is right or wrong when conflicting information arises. There are poorly done (and published) systematic reviews, and there are well-informed experts. Experts are often right (that is why they are experts), but the potential for bias is high. Objective and forthright experts are easily identified and develop a reputation for minimizing and acknowledging their biases. For busy clinicians, these unbiased experts are immensely valuable resources. In contrast, systematic reviews and randomized controlled trials (RCTs) can be wrong, or poorly

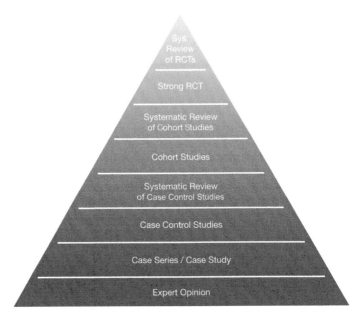

Fig. 1. A hierarchy of evidence for clinical dental research. This hierarchy is best understood as a risk for bias pyramid, not a hierarchy of truth. The higher levels of evidence are more likely to be correct, but they are not implicitly superior. Sys, systematic.

done, or grossly overinterpreted, although they are less likely to be wrong because of biases. The hierarchy is best understood to represent the potential for biases affecting the resulting recommendations, so perhaps a reliability pyramid is a better term for them. Every study has inherent biases. The best studies recognize this, apply analytical and study design techniques to mitigate them, and acknowledge how they may have affected the results and conclusions.

In brief, a systematic review (preferably with a meta-analysis) attempts to answer a question (eg, do screw-retained implant crowns survive longer than cemented implant crowns?) by aggregating, synthesizing, and analyzing all relevant published studies. Clinicians might consider it an expert-level book report. It is an attempt to analyze the existing data in a meaningful way. This approach only works if there are sufficient studies on a given topic, and its resultant quality depends on the quality of the included studies. The systematic review is a report on the current preponderance of evidence, which is the metric by which clinical decisions are best made.

Anecdotally, it seems there has been a strong trend in clinical dentistry to publish and cite (formally or casually) systematic reviews. Although I appreciate the enthusiasm for increased levels of evidence, clinicians need to think about systematic reviews for a moment.

Systematic reviews should be performed by a group of experts knowledgeable in the field. Such undertakings require deep understanding of the problem at hand, which questions need to be asked, which studies should be included, and how to properly interpret the results. Such tasks are not best performed in the early stages of a career.

Not all systematic reviews are created equal, and in clinical dentistry this is especially true. **Table 1** shows that the position of systematic reviews in the hierarchy depends on the types (and quality) of the studies analyzed. Systematic reviews built on less rigorous studies are not at the top of the pyramid.

Table 1
Levels of evidence for clinical treatment disciplines

Study Design	What It Is	Relevance to Clinical Dentistry
Systematic reviews of homogenous RCTs	An expert synthesis of the best available interventions on a particular topic	This is the highest level of evidence. However, rarely seen in clinical disciplines because of the sparsity of strong RCTs
Strong RCTs	A random, controlled, blinded trial. The only way to establish cause and effect	Rare in any surgical discipline (especially clinical dentistry). Best available new evidence
Systematic review of cohort studies	An expert synthesis of the best available observational studies	Good for summarizing risk factors associated with an outcome
Individual cohort studies	A high-level observational study. No treatment is performed on patients as part of the study	In general, a tool used less in clinical dentistry and more in the public health disciplines and epidemiology
Systematic review of case control studies	An expert synthesis of the best available research for risk factors for rare outcomes	Not common in clinical dentistry
Case control studies	A cross-sectional study used to identify risk factors for rare outcomes	An efficient way to identify risks for diseases not often seen
Case series	A series of cases showing proof of concept. Not proof of expected results or expected complications	Useful in seeing what might be possible by experts. Useful for exploring new techniques or materials. Interpret cautiously
Expert opinion	A well-regarded individual's or group's opinion on a topic. Reliability and accuracy depend on the veracity and knowledge of the expert	Efficient and practical method for finding information. High risk potential for bias

However, in clinical dentistry (and in surgical medical fields), clinicians have a problem: the best novel evidence is a sufficiently powered RCT (**Fig. 2**) with narrow variation in the results. High-quality RCTs are expensive to execute and require strong management, oversight, and analysis. Randomizing patients into control or placebo groups in clinical treatment produces ethical and practical challenges (is anyone interested in a placebo surgery?). Blinding of patients, operators, and evaluators is nearly impossible for obvious reasons. In addition, even when such challenges are addressed, recruitment of sufficient numbers of participants commonly proves problematic. As a result, there are not enough RCTs of any quality in clinical dentistry,

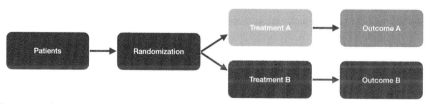

Fig. 2. Randomized clinical trial design.

let alone high-quality RCTs. Much of what is commonly published in the dental literature as RCTs are often better classified as clinical trials because of a lack of true
randomization, controls, and blinding. A clinical trial is essentially a large, more
rigorous case series with quantified analysis.

There are various methodological approaches to creating a systematic review.
Among the most well regarded is the Cochrane Review. The rigor of the Cochrane
approach synthesizes the appropriate studies into concise and reliable results. Only
high-quality studies are included in such reviews. However, clinical dental research
is not well funded, and clinicians do not see many high-quality clinical studies for
any given question. As a result, a highly rigorous Cochrane Review for a given clinical
dental technique or device often produces conclusions such as, "The quality of the evidence is assessed as very low due to high and unclear risk of bias of primary studies
and there is some evidence of reporting bias so clinicians should treat these findings
with caution."[1] Although honest, this is not very useful when clinicians are looking for
scientific guidance to treat their patients. The high rigor of the Cochrane Reviews often
leaves practitioners in clinical dentistry without much guidance.

As such, many systematic reviews published in clinical dentistry do not adhere to
the Cochrane guidelines and use other, less restrictive frameworks in order to find
something useful to say about the evidence. This approach produces more clinically
relevant information but with a higher risk for errors and bias. Imagine a systematic review with strong conclusion and recommendation statements finding that immediate
loading of implants is highly successful. On the surface, this seems to be a high-level
recommendation about what success rates can be expected with this procedure.
However, what if the systematic review was built on 4 small case series, 2 of which
were from 1 author, and all of which were performed by experts? It is easy to see
how such conclusions might be biased toward results that will not prove generalizable.

Cohort studies are nonintervention studies; they are observational exclusively. This
term is commonly misused in published titles in dentistry. They are not useful for determining what techniques or materials perform better. They are used to see how risk factors affect an outcome. For example, Raes and colleagues[2] studied 2 groups of
implant patients over time: smokers and nonsmokers. The primary outcome being
evaluated was papilla regeneration, for which the smoking group was at significantly
greater risk to not regenerate papilla.

Case control studies are also strictly observational. They are designed to find associated risk factors for a rare outcome. The resulting odds ratio indicates the odds of a
patient with the risk factor developing the disease outcome. For example, Becker and
colleagues[3] studied the effect of osteoporosis on the odds of having an implant failure.
This exploratory study was unable to find any association between osteoporosis and
implant failure. This finding does not mean that there is no real association. There may
be, but perhaps it is too small to see with this sample size, or perhaps there is too
much variation. These issues are discussed later. The results of observational studies
are correlation only and do not prove causation, but they may hint at it.

The case series and case study mostly commonly reside near the bottom of every
hierarchy of evidence, but why then are they so frequently published in many high-
level clinical dental journals? As a procedural discipline, clinical dentistry relies heavily
on advancement in techniques and protocols to improve outcomes. Such develop-
ments are difficult or impossible to test in RCTs and observational studies. Case series
and case studies come in various levels of rigor and reliability. At the most rigorous
end, the case series is designed with a primary outcome measurement (eg, number
of prosthetic complications with angled screw channels). The next (n) number of participants (n) is determined in advance, along with strict inclusion/exclusion criteria. The

next (n) number of patients to present to the clinics, willing to participate, and meeting the inclusion criteria are included in the study. The outcome (complications) is tracked for each and the results analyzed. There is no control or alternative group with which they will be compared. Where appropriate, the results can be cautiously compared with values obtained from other studies (historical control). If performed and reported honestly, the rigorous case series can provide ideas about short-term or intraoperative complications and results.

The case study (sometimes called a clinical report) is similar to the case series but much less rigorous. The case study is simply a qualitative presentation of 1 to several similar cases (sometimes mistakenly published with "case series" in the title to appear more rigorous). The included cases are selected solely by the investigators (beware of selection bias). There are no comparisons to be made and there is no accounting for how these patients were selected and others not. In general, a case study (or weak case series) is best regarded as the best of what is possible by the author. The results may not be generalizable to other clinicians or patient populations, nor may they be predictable. It could be imagined that a clinician performed the same procedure hundreds of times with mediocre results, but in a few instances the outcomes were outstanding. Only those few outstanding cases make the article, and no analysis is performed to see what the normal results were and how divergent the outcomes may have been. The case study is a proof-of-concept study, a sample of what might be possible. For example, Schoenbaum and colleagues[4] showed resolution of peri-implant gingival recession by the use of an interim restoration. This approach is proof only of what is possible and may not indicate what is common.

INTRODUCTION TO BIOSTATISTICS

In the remainder of this article, the intention is not to turn readers into biostatisticians, nor would they even be interested. It is the job of the journals, and their review teams, to ensure that the proper study design and analyses were performed. The better the journal, the more rigorous they are about this process. Nor does this article explain how a trial should be set up or which tests should or should not be performed. However, it may help clinicians become better consumers (and critics) of the published dental literature.

Bias

In particular, this article focuses on publication bias. By the time an article is published, a bias in selection has been made at several different levels: demographics of patients seeking this treatment, clinicians so proficient they intend to publish their results, cases worthy of publication, results the author wants to publish, and results the editor wants in the journal. Each of these biases contributes to published results that generally do not indicate what might happen on average. For example, it could easily be imagined that investigators and editors would have little interest in publishing a study looking for (and failing to detect) a correlation between selective serotonin reuptake inhibitors (SSRIs) and implant failure. It is not very interesting to report that here is yet another factor that has no effect on failure. Imagine 30 such studies were performed. If the threshold for significance is $P<.05$, it should be expected that, through nothing but chance alone, at least 1 of those studies would find a "significant" correlation between SSRIs and implant failure. This study is the one that will be published. The data from the other 29 will not. This situation is analogous to the multiple testing error in statistics, but on a metascale secondary to publication bias.[5]

Statistical Significance or Clinical Significance

When skimming an article, clinicians often look for the results table and look for the variables that have an asterisk or boldface indicating $P<.05$. They conclude that this variable is important and the others are not. The late Paulo Vigolo[6] published an excellent 10-year RCT examining whether splinting adjacent implant restorations in the posterior maxilla maintains better bone levels than nonsplinted restorations (the controls). At the 10-year follow-up of 114 implant restorations, he found a statistically significant difference in bone levels between splinted and nonsplinted groups. The splinted restoration design preserved "significantly" more bone ($P = .0042$) than the nonsplinted group. If the discussion was stopped there, the understanding of this study would lead to the conclusion that restorations should be splinted in an effort to preserve peri-implant bone. A closer analysis reveals that, although the effect is present, it might hardly be considered a strong enough effect to suggest splinting for this reason. The effect at 10 years was that splinted restorations preserved 0.1 mm more bone. As Dr Vigolo wisely noted in this article: "A significant difference in bone loss was seen between the two groups. However, the difference of 0.1 mm [at 10 years] was not considered clinically meaningful."[6] Statistical significance does not equal clinical significance. Statistical significance (ie, $P<.05$) indicates that an effect is likely present, but clinical significance indicates whether it is relevant.

Forest Plots

One of the most reliable and efficient ways to find strong scientific evidence for clinical questions is a well-done systematic review with a meta-analysis. The output of the meta-analysis is called a forest plot, which is a summary graphic of results of all studies included in the review. The ability to quickly interpret a forest plot is essential to quickly getting an overall look at the data for the question at hand. When a comparison is being made between 2 groups (eg, cement-retained crowns and screw-retained crowns; **Fig. 3**), the vertical bar in the middle represents the line of no difference between groups. The purple squares represent the weight allotted to the study (usually from sample size). The horizontal lines (usually) represent the 95%

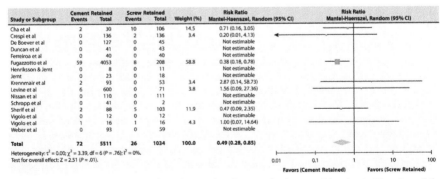

Fig. 3. Forest plot comparison of studies evaluating survival rates of implants. The size of the purple square reflects its weight in the analysis; green diamond is the overall results of the meta-analysis. CI, confidence interval. (*From* Lemos CA, de Souza Batista VE, de Faria Almeida DA, et al. Evaluation of cement-retained versus screw-retained implant-supported restorations for marginal bone loss: A systematic review and meta-analysis. J Prosth Dent. 2016;115:424; with permission.)

confidence interval (CI) of that study. Shorter horizontal bars indicate greater precision or consistency in the results. The green diamond at the bottom is the overall effect estimated based on the included studies. The example from Lemos and colleagues[7] (see **Fig. 3**) indicates that cemented restorations show a significant (and clinically significant) reduction in peri-implant bone loss. However, as with many clinical dental meta-analyses, the CIs for each study are huge and most studies have small sample sizes.[7] Most of the results of this particular analysis are skewed by the result from 1 study[8], which had many more participants than any other. Interpretation of such data should be cautious.

Interpreting Graphs

When reviewing graphs in the literature (and especially in product marketing), special attention should be given to the units and the scale of the graphs. Is the scale in 1-mm increments or 0.1 mm? Does the scale start at 0 or some number to emphasize effect? **Fig. 4** shows the same hypothetical data presented with 2 different scales. One implies a huge difference between groups, whereas the other minimizes this impression. There is no right or wrong way to display the data, except that it should be done with an honest intent to show the results.

Confidence Intervals

CIs represent a key method to show the precision of a measurement. If continuous data are used (ie, numeric value measurements), the mean is only part of what clinicians should want to know. The precision of the values that provide that mean is also important. It is an oversimplification, but the 95% CI is best understood to mean that there is a 95% chance that the true mean for the group lies within this range. Samples that have more consistent results have a narrower CI for the group. For example, if there are 2 types of implants both with a mean implant stability quotient (ISQ) at an insertion of 72, they might be imagined to be comparable. However, what if group A had all values between 68 and 76, whereas group B had values spread between 55 and 80? Group A clearly has much greater consistency and predictability for ISQ compared with group B. This dataset could be presented as:

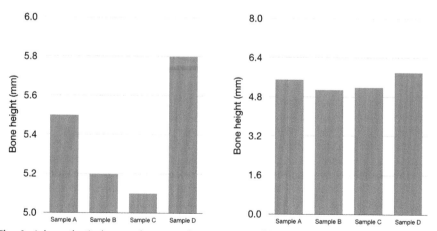

Fig. 4. A hypothetical example comparing 4 groups of bone graft materials. The data are the same in both groups. Alteration of the y-axis scale produces very different impressions about the differences between groups.

Mean ISQ (95% CI)
Group A = 72 (70–74)
Group B = 72 (61–75)

Power and Sample Size

Unfortunately, clinically relevant dental research is woefully underfunded. This situation is not likely to change anytime soon. Therefore, clinicians must often to try to understand what to expect clinically from limited or highly variable data. It is an unfortunate reality for the profession.

The sample sizes are often too small. There is no preset number of samples that makes a study useful (eg, n = 10 or n = 100). The size of the sample needed depends on the difference that is expected to be seen between groups, the variability within groups, and the precision desired. A nondental example: imagine investigators want to determine the true difference in mean mass between golden retrievers and Labradors. There is probably a difference, but previous data have shown that it is not much, maybe 1 kg. A large number of dogs (maybe 1000) will be needed from each breed to find a statistically significant difference. If instead investigators want to find whether there is a difference in weights between house cats and bull mastiffs, they would need very few from each group to find a statistically significant difference (maybe n = 5).

If investigators intend to find a difference between groups, they need a sufficient number of samples for each group, and that number depends on the expected size of the difference. To see small differences, large sample sizes are needed, whereas large differences require much smaller samples sizes. This idea is an important part of power calculations. Power is the chance that a difference can be seen between groups (based on an estimate of the means, variability, and sample size). The biostatistical norm is to use 80% as the power threshold, meaning that there will be an 80% chance to see a difference, and a 20% chance of not being able to see the difference even when there is a difference. Power analyses are generally used to determine the number of samples needed in each group. If there are too few samples, the study is underpowered. There is an increased likelihood that no statistically significant difference will be seen between the groups, even though there really is a difference.

Overinterpretation

Clinicians must synthesize the results of multiple questions and concerns for every decision they make. One part of that process is the scientific data with which they are familiar. The more informed clinicians are in a discipline, the better the decisions will be. As clinicians begin their journey of incorporating science into their practices, they must keep in mind that each study is only a piece of the overall puzzle. A single study is not conclusive evidence. It is but 1 piece, of a mountain of data, answering only 1 question. Each decision requires answers to multiple questions, and each question has dozens (it is hoped) of studies attempting to provide answers. There will be conflicting data. There will be questions that have superior results for group A, and other questions that will have superior results for group B. Part of being (or becoming) the best that clinicians can be is understanding those differences and making the appropriate choices given conflicting information. Do not look at a single study and assume its results represent the definitive answer to that single question, and certainly not to all the questions that clinicians must answer.

I would also like to briefly explain the difference between efficacy and effectiveness. When studies are performed by experts, in highly controlled environments, with carefully selected and informed patients, the results are in the category of efficacy. When clinicians treat patients in busy clinical practices, with patients that are not as carefully selected, informed, or controlled, this is in the category of effectiveness. The complications, and success rates, of these 2 environments are very different. Do not assume that the results obtained in a published study de facto represent what clinicians see in clinical practice. Efficacy represents the best of what might be possible given every factor is tuned to the highest levels.

SUMMARY

Exceptional clinicians rely on the best available evidence. The data in clinical dentistry are sometimes insufficient and flawed. However, some data are better than no data. The better prepared clinicians are to understand the science and see the benefits and limitations, the better prepared they are for improving the quality of care. Those who are striving toward excellence must insist on scientific data, and should themselves be working to contribute.

DISCLOSURE

The author has nothing to disclose.

REFERENCES

1. Esposito M, Grusovin MG, Maghaireh H, et al. Interventions for replacing missing teeth: different times for loading dental implants. Cochrane Database Syst Rev 2013;(3):CD003878.
2. Raes S, Rocci A, Raes F, et al. A prospective cohort study on the impact of smoking on soft tissue alterations around single implants. Clin Oral Implants Res 2015; 26(9):1086–90.
3. Becker W, Hujoel PP, Becker BE, et al. Osteoporosis and implant failure: an exploratory case-control study. J Periodontol 2000;71:625–31.
4. Schoenbaum TR, Solnit GS, Alawie S, et al. Treatment of peri-implant recession with a screw-retained, interim implant restoration: A clinical report. J Prosthet Dent 2019;121:212–6.
5. Ioannidis JP. Why most discovered true associations are inflated. J Epidemiol 2008;19:640–8.
6. Vigolo P, Mutinelli S, Zaccaria M, et al. Clinical evaluation of marginal bone level change around multiple adjacent implants restored with splinted and nonsplinted restorations: a 10-year randomized controlled trial. Int J Oral Maxillofac Implants 2015;30:411–8.
7. Lemos CA, de Souza Batista VE, de Faria Almeida DA, et al. Evaluation of cement-retained versus screw-retained implant-supported restorations for marginal bone loss: A systematic review and meta-analysis. J Prosthet Dent 2016;115:419–27.
8. Fugazzotto PA, Vlassis J, Butler B. ITI implant use in private practice: clinical results with 5,526 implants followed up to 72+ months in function. Int J Oral Maxillofac Implants 2004;19(3):408–12.

FURTHER READINGS

Burns PB, Rohrich RJ, Chung KC. The levels of evidence and their role in evidence-based medicine. Plast Reconstr Surg 2011;128:305.
Del Fabbro G, Bzovsky S, Thoma A, et al. Hierarchy of evidence in surgical research. In: Thoma A, editor. Evidence-based surgery. Cham (Switzerland): Springer; 2019. p. 37–49.
Motulsky H. Essential biostatistics: a nonmathematical approach. New York: Oxford University Press; 2015.

Review of the Modern Dental Ceramic Restorative Materials for Esthetic Dentistry in the Minimally Invasive Age

Alireza Moshaverinia, DDS, MS, PhD

KEYWORDS

• Ceramics • Dental materials • Dental ceramics

KEY POINTS

- Material selection is among the most important decisions to be made by clinicians; proper material selection can affect the long-term function, longevity, and esthetics of restorations.
- The large number of restorative material have provided great number of choices for restorative dentists, but has increased the complexity of the decision-making process.
- The overwhelming number of restorative dental materials mean that improper material selection can potentially lead to failures in the outcome.
- This article provides the practitioner with up-to-date practical information on ceramic restorative materials and techniques and decision-making guides to help determine the best ceramic material for various clinical scenarios.

INTRODUCTION

In modern restorative dentistry, we are overwhelmed with a plethora of different ceramic restorative materials available in dental market, which makes the process of material selection very confusing for a restorative dentist. Increased patient concerns about esthetics have led to widespread use of dental ceramic materials. Restorative dentists are bombarded with so much information from dental manufacturers and their representatives that it sometimes makes the selection criteria for different clinical scenarios were complicated. It is very well-known that achieving successful clinical outcomes are attributed with 2 important factors: (1) knowledge of dental material and selection of the correct dental material and (2) the hand skills of the practitioner, including proper handling of the dental material and proper communication with

The author has nothing to disclose.
Division of Advanced Prosthodontics, UCLA School of Dentistry, 10833 Leconte Avenue, B3-023 CHS, Los Angeles, CA 90095-1668, USA
E-mail address: amoshaverinia@ucla.edu

Dent Clin N Am 64 (2020) 621–631
https://doi.org/10.1016/j.cden.2020.05.002

dental.theclinics.com

the laboratory technician. With this combination we are able to deliver proper restorations to our patients in a routine bases.

Here, it has been attempted to simplify this confusion in the selection of ceramic dental materials. A systematic approach and a decision-making guide will be provided to help the restorative dentist choose the best material in each clinical situation.

WHAT ARE DENTAL CERAMICS?

A ceramic is a product made from a nonmetallic inorganic material that is processed by firing at high temperature to achieve desirable mechanical and optical properties. The development of ceramic dental restorative materials as a metal-free category of restoratives has been a milestone in treatment options that changed the clinical workflow of dentists.[1,2] The technical improvements in development of ceramic materials have enabled scientists to marry the impeccable advantages of ceramics such as excellent esthetic appearance and optical properties with superior biocompatibility, improved mechanical properties, and low plaque retention.[3,4] To be used in everyday dentistry, ceramics need to meet specific criteria: (1) appropriate toughness—the material needs to be tough and withstand crack propagation, (2) suitable mechanical strength to withstand occlusal forces, (3) favorable optical and desirable esthetic properties, and (4) predictable in vivo performance offering long-lasting and durable restorations.

Generally, we expect dental ceramics to be translucent at incisal edges, opacious at cervical edges, provide adequate strength, and enable conservation of tooth structure. Owing to excellent esthetic and prosthetic properties, ceramics could be used as a framework material in all types of tooth restorations, including single crowns, inlays or onlays, and laminate veneers.[5,6] The presence of different phases in the ceramic composition along with manufacturing processes have provided the dentists with an array of restorative materials to choose. Broadly speaking, dental ceramics could be classified into the following broad categories to help clinicians select the best material based on their patients need: glassy ceramics, resin matrix ceramics, and polycrystalline ceramics.[7,8] In light of this, a brief overview of this classification will be given in the following sections to shed more light on the properties and functionality of dental ceramic materials.

Glass Matrix Ceramics

These nonmetallic inorganic multiphase ceramics are usually composed of a residual glass phase with finely dispersed crystalline phases.[8,9] The glassy ceramics are usually fabricated by precise crystallization of the glass nucleated evenly throughout the glass phase or by embedding 1 or more crystals in the structure.[10,11] The crystallin phase can occupy 0.5% to 99.0% of the composition, but usually contains 30% to 70% of the final composition.[11] The type, size, and volume fraction of the crystallin phase along with its distribution in the glass matrix are among the important factors controlling the mechanical and aesthetic properties, such as the toughness and translucency of the final material. Moreover, the presence of crystallin phase improves the mechanical strength of the final material by inhibiting crack propagation and growth.[12] The glassy phase also contributes to the improved mechanical properties by filling the grain boundaries. The advantage of glass matrix ceramics over traditional ceramics include ease of synthesis processes, less shrinkage, improved translucency owing to the decreased internal light scattering.[13,14] The glass matrix ceramics are generally divided into 2 subcategories: natural materials such as Feldspathic ceramics and synthetic materials such as lithium disilicate.

Feldspathic ceramics

The feldspar-based ceramics are known as the traditional dental ceramics based on a ternary system composed of natural feldspars (potassium/sodium aluminosilicate), Kaolin ($Al_2O_3.SiO_2.2H_2O$), quartz (SiO_2), and some metal oxides as additives.[10] During the fabrication process, the melting feldspar provides a glassy matrix for distribution of a disordered network of silica tetrahedra. The improved strength of potassium containing feldspars known as leucite ($K_2Al_2Si_6O_{16}$) turn them into a suitable option for veneering material on metal and ceramic substrates or as reinforced resin-bonded glass-ceramic cores. This class of glass ceramic dental restorative material can be produced in different tooth shades with a range of opacity and translucency by adding different metal oxide pigments. In routine dentistry, the opaque feldspar ceramics are used as a first layer shielding the underlying metal followed by a layer of enamel ceramics to develop the natural color of the tooth. Despite the advantageous properties, feldspathic porcelains are limited to low load-bearing anterior applications owing to lesser flexural strength and increased brittleness. The perceived color of natural teeth is the result of the reflectance from the dentin modified by the absorption, scattering, and thickness of the enamel.[1] One of the primary factors that influences the appearance of layered ceramic restorations is the layering effect. Translucent porcelain may have a greater effect on the color of the veneered restoration than the opaque substrate. There is a significant correlation between the thickness ratio of core and veneer ceramics and the color of the restoration. Even when adequate ceramic thickness exists, clinical shade matches are difficult to achieve, because there is a wide range of translucency among the core materials of all-ceramic systems at clinically relevant core thicknesses. Clinicians claim that porcelain of high opacity should be used to decrease the perceived color difference of porcelain veneers after bonding to dark or discolored tooth substances. Different manufacturers have introduced porcelain systems with increased opacity and claim superior color stability over different backgrounds. Layered feldspathic veneers are indicated when restoring tetracycline tooth or discolored preparations owing to the fact that layered porcelain powders gives more flexibility with respect to choice of opacity and translucent areas. Further, layered feldspathic veneers are indicated when undertaking more conservative cases in younger population with large pulps owing to the fact that less tooth structure needs to be removed. Many dentists choose feldspathic veneers because they can be made thinner than pressed ceramic with more than 1 color of porcelain throughout the veneer. Vitablocs (Vita Zahnfabrik, Bad Säckingen, Germany) are among the most used feldspar-based computer-aided drafting/computer-aided manufacturing ceramics with an average flexural strength of 154 MPa.

Lithium disilicate

The synthetic glass ceramics have emerged as an alternative to become independent of the natural resources and their inherent variations with higher volume fraction of crystallin phase distributed in a glassy matrix. Currently, lithium disilicate glass ceramics are among the popular restorative dental materials that are available as heat-pressable ingot and a partially crystallized machinable block.[15] Lithium disilicate glass-ceramics are one of the well-known synthetic glass-ceramics based on SiO_2–Li_2O system composed of randomly oriented fine platelet-like or rod-like entangled lithium disilicate crystals at higher concentrations of up to 70% and a lower concentration of lithium orthophosphate (Li_3PO_4) crystals heterogeneously dispersed in the glass matrix.[10,13] The higher concentration of crystallin phase and the tighter interlocking matrix of this synthetic glass ceramic poses significantly higher strength of approximately 350 MPa and fracture toughness of 2.5 MPa m$^{1/2}$ compared with the naturally occurring feldspathic porcelain.[13,16] Secondary to the improved mechanical properties, this restorative material can have a wide range of applications including resin-bonded veneers, crowns, and 3-unit bridges up to the second premolar. IPS e.max (Ivoclar Vivadent, Schaan, Liechtenstein), a lithium disilicate ceramic, was developed in part by Prof. Wolfram Holland at Ivoclar Vivadent. After the development of clinical applications, the material was released to the dental community about 12 years ago. This ceramic material is well-researched, and many authors have described its physical properties. The effect that flaws in IPS e.max lithium disilicate or luting agent spaces have on fracture potential and tensile strength have been tested, as well as the effects of physiologic aging in a water environment, abrasiveness, wear, and surface roughness. It has met, or exceeded, almost all of the clinical requirements considered ideal for a dental ceramic used in clinical practice.

Celtra Duo (Dentsply Sirona, York, PA) is one of the newly available lithium silicate-based ceramics available in the market. It is a zirconia-reinforced lithium silicate with the amount of Zr inclusion is around 10% zirconium oxide. The manufacturer claims that the smaller ceramic crystal size and ultrafine microstructure material lead to increased mechanical strength. Celtra Duo lithium silicate-based ceramics are available in pressable or milled formats and can be used crowns and bonded partial crowns (inlays, onlays, and veneers).[17]

The other lithium silicate-based ceramics is GC Initial LiSi Press (GC America, Alsip, IL), which is a high-strength and high-density lithium disilicate-based ceramic. This new lithium silicate ceramic offers equal distribution of microcrystals, leading to excellent mechanical and optical properties. The recommended indications for this pressable ceramics are crowns, inlays, onlays, veneers and 3-unit fixed partial dentures up to the second premolar.[18]

Resin Matrix Ceramics

A generalized definition of a resin matrix ceramic is a hybrid material composed of an organic matrix highly filled with inorganic particles such as ceramics, glasses, and glass ceramics.[19] The polymer matric provides a supportive network reinforcing the inorganic network of the hybrid material. The American Dental Association Code on Dental Procedures and Nomenclature used to exclude the resin matrix material from being classified as ceramic materials; however, its 2013 version defined the term ceramic as "pressed, fired, polished, or milled materials containing predominantly inorganic refractory compounds - including porcelains, glasses, ceramics, and glass-ceramics."[20] Therefore, the resin matrix hybrids fall into dental ceramics category because they contain more than 50% inorganic particles. This class of dental materials are a suitable choice for computer-aided drafting/computer-aided manufacturing, providing superior properties compared with the traditional ceramics and glass ceramics such as better mimicking the elasticity of dentin and ease of milling and adjusting.[8]

Polycrystalline Ceramics

This class of dental restoratives are nonmetallic inorganic all ceramic materials without any glassy phase.[8] The fine grain crystals tightly arranged into regular arrays by directly sintering the crystals in the absence of any intervening material that promotes the strength of the material by reducing crack propagation.[9] Despite improved mechanical properties, the polycrystalline ceramics have limited translucency. One approach to enhance the translucency is to reduce the light scattering through decreasing number of grain boundaries by increasing the grain size.[1] However, increasing the crystallin grain size can result in reduction of mechanical properties.

In addition, etching the polycrystalline ceramics with hydrofluoric acid seems to be very difficult owing to absence of the glass phase. Aluminum oxide (Alumina) and Zirconia are among the popular polycrystalline ceramics that will be discussed briefly in the following subsections.

Alumina

Alumina (Al_2O_3) is a natural metal oxide with a broad range of industrial applications such as abrasive materials secondary to its high hardness. Besides higher hardness, the superior wear and corrosion resistance along with biocompatibility have turned this material into a popular candidate in dentistry.[21] The very fine grain size of medical-grade alumina ceramics hinders static fatigue and deflects cracks while under load. All these properties have turned Alumina into a desirable substrate for a wide range of medical applications, including dental restoratives and orthopedic applications. However, the Alumina ceramics are prone to bulk fractures owing to higher elasticity.[22] Procera AllCeram from Nobel Biocare (Zürich, Switzerland) (the first fully dense polycrystalline ceramic) and In-Ceram AL, a product of VITA Zahnfabrik, are representatives of this type of ceramic.

Zirconia

Zirconia (zirconium dioxide) is a polycrystalline ceramic with excellent toughness, strength, and fatigue resistance. Depending on the temperature, this polymorphic ceramic can be formed in 3 different crystallographic phases as cubic forming at temperatures of more than 2300°C, tetragonal occurring at temperatures between 1100°C and 2300°C, and monoclinic phase occurring at room temperatures to 1100°C.[23,24] Zirconia has an elasticity similar to stainless steel, but superior biocompatibility. In addition, the decreased plaque retention results in healthier gums after application of zirconia.[25] Zirconia restorations continue to be successful (from the standpoint of fit, retention, wear, and fracture resistance), and yet controversial in some clinical leader and academic circles, for use in simple single unit and more complex restorations. There are perhaps 50 different zirconia ceramics on the market and, often, the laboratory technician or clinician have no idea what the manufacturing standards were for a given zirconia block or disk used to fabricate restorations coming from different sources. The physical strength and ability to resist fatigue fracture depends on the manufacturing standard that is applied by a specific manufacturer. Yttria-stabilized zirconia (with flexural strength of >900 MPa) is indicated for clinical situations including anterior and posterior crowns, implant abutments/crowns, 3-unit inlay and onlay bridges, cantilever bridges with a minimum of 2 abutment teeth and a maximum of 1 pontic of no more than 1 premolar width, and multiunit long span (up to 14 units)

MATERIAL SELECTION TREE

Fig. 1. Ceramic dental materials selection tree showing the important parameters to consider before ceramic material selection in different clinical scenarios.

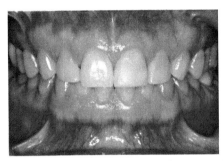
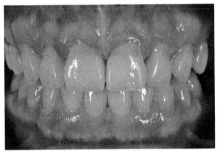

Fig. 2. (*Left*) Preoperative view of patient's frontal intraoral view. Patient specifically requesting change of the restorations of her anterior maxillary sextant without losing any of her tooth structure. (*Right*) Intraoral frontal view of the definitive feldspathic ceramic restorations. Please note that lithium disilicate ceramics could also be used in this clinical case. (*Courtesy of* Mr. Domenico Cascione, BS, CDT, MDT, Santa Monica, California.)

(DC-Zircon). Some of the available zirconia dental ceramics such as Lava Plus High Translucency Zirconia (3M ESPE, St Paul, MN) are indicated for clinical circumstances with limited interocclusal space, in addition to situations when the tooth-preserving preparation is needed where minimum of 0.5 mm occlusal wall thickness is available.[2] The flexural strength of widely used zirconia dental ceramics range from 1.0 to 1.4 GPa (Glidewell [Newport Beach, CA] BruxZir Solid Zirconia, 1–1.4 GPa; Ivoclar Vivadent Zenostar T, 1.2 GPa; Katana Zirconia [Kuraray Noritake Dental Inc., Okayama, Japan]).

Owing to their high opacity, several studies have tried to enhance the translucency of the zirconia materials by modification of their microstructure, including decreasing the alumina content, increasing the density, decreasing the grain size, adding cubic phase zirconia, and decreasing the amount of impurities and structural defects.[2] The size of the crystalline grain is the microstructural feature that is more closely related to the adjustment of the translucency of polycrystalline ceramics. The creation of ceramic materials with high translucency has been done in the past by means of increasing the grain size during sintering. Larger grains lead to a smaller number of grain boundaries, thereby decreasing light scattering. For Y-TZP, it has been shown

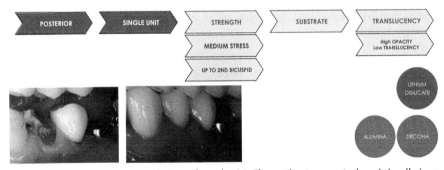

Fig. 3. (*Left*) Preoperative lateral view of tooth #21. The patient requested a minimally invasive approach to preserve his tooth structure (no full coverage crowns). (*Right*) Definitive bonded lithium disilicate ceramic restoration. Please note that feldspathic porcelain is contraindicated in this clinical situation. Alternative ceramic material options are mention on the right side corner.

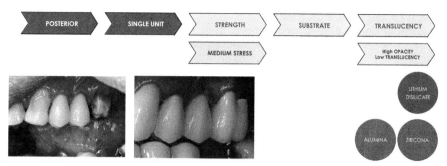

Fig. 4. (*Left*) Preoperative lateral view of tooth #14. (*Right*) Definitive zirconia ceramic restoration. Alternative ceramic material options are mention on the right side corner.

that larger grains are detrimental for both the mechanical properties and the stability of the tetragonal phase. Therefore, the translucency of zirconia cannot be achieved by means of increasing its grain size. The increased translucency made the zirconia ceramic materials slightly more esthetic, but it was challenging for laboratory technician to achieve esthetic outcomes consistently.

An alternative method to fabricate high translucent Y-TZP is achieved by decreasing the grain size significantly. Nevertheless, the grain size needs to be decreased until reaching a critical value that results in mitigation of the so-called birefringence phenomenon.[4] Birefringence occurs in Y-TZP owing to the large amount of tetragonal crystal phase (>90%), which is a crystal that has different refractive indexes according to its crystallographic orientation in the microstructure. Such anisotropic behavior related to the variation in the refractive index causes significant light scattering. Another way to overcome these scattering effects is the use of cubic zirconia, which offers optical isotropic behavior, increasing the translucency.[2] These newer, highly translucent zirconia materials are certainly more translucent than the original monolithic zirconia dental ceramic materials. However, increased translucency (owing to increase in cubic structure content) causes a decrease in the flexural strength. The flexural strength of highly translucent zirconia ranges from 500 to 800 MPa (Glidewell BruxZir Anterior and Ivoclar Weiland Zenostar MT, and Katana [Noritake] STML, 750 MPa and UTML 560 MPa). It has been reported that the translucency of zirconia is variable depending on the processing method, manufacturer formulation, and laboratory sintering times and temperatures.

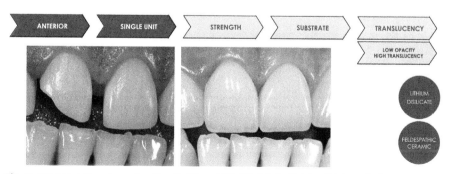

Fig. 5. Preoperative view of patient's #8 and #9. (*Right*) Definitive lithium disilicate ceramic restorations. Please note that feldspathic porcelain could also be used in this clinical case.

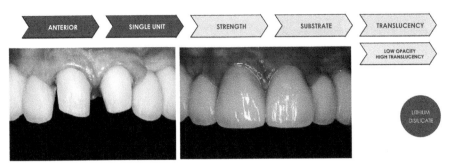

Fig. 6. (*Left*) Preoperative view of patient's #8 and #9. (*Right*) Definitive lithium disilicate ceramic restorations. Ceramic material was selected based on substrate percentage of enamel and dentin.

CASE SELECTION AND CLINICAL CONSIDERATIONS (MATERIAL SELECTION)

In this article, we have reviewed some of the widely used dental ceramic materials in the market and discussing their mechanical, optical, and handling properties. Here, a material selection (**Fig. 1**) tree is provided to help the clinician and restorative dentist to choose the appropriate type of restorative material in different clinical scenarios.

To select the suitable type of ceramic dental material, there are important parameters to be considered:

1. Position: The clinician should consider the fact that the restoration will be used in as an anterior or posterior restoration. For anterior restorations (**Fig. 2**) a more translucent ceramic material with lower mechanical strength lead to favorable esthetic outcomes. However, for posterior restoration where translucency is not of importance a stronger ceramic material such as alumina, zirconia, or bonded lithium disilicate are indicated (**Figs. 3** and **4**).
2. Design: The clinician should consider the design of the ceramic restoration: single unit versus splinted. Definitely for multiple splinted unit restorations, a stronger ceramic material is recommended.
3. Strength: A biomechanical risk assessment is necessary to analyze the amounts of expected occlusal forces. For a low to medium biomechanical stresses, feldspathic

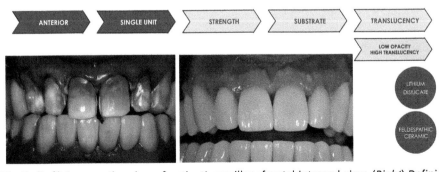

Fig. 7. (*Left*) Preoperative view of patient's maxillary frontal intraoral view. (*Right*) Definitive lithium disilicate ceramic restorations. Please note that feldspathic porcelain could also be used in this clinical case; however, masking the discolored teeth and percentage of dentin are not favorable factors for feldspathic porcelain application.

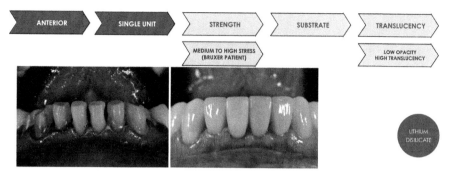

Fig. 8. (*Left*) Preoperative view of patient's mandibular frontal intraoral view. The patient reports a history of nocturnal bruxism, but still wanted veneers. (*Right*) Definitive lithium disilicate ceramic restorations. Please note that feldspathic porcelain might not be desirable alternative ceramic restorative material owing to discolored substrate teeth, low percentage of enamel of substrate, and unfavorable biomechanical assessment.

or lithium disilicate ceramics are recommended. However, for more medium to high amounts of occlusal stresses, stronger ceramics such as alumina or zirconia are indicated (see **Fig. 4**).

4. Substrate: The tooth or material substrate is one of the most important selection criteria for ceramic restorative materials. There are 3 factors to take into account: percentage of enamel left, percentage of dentin left, and presence or absence of discoloration. The presence of enamel and dentin favors a ceramic material that can be reliably bonded to tooth structure, such as feldspathic porcelain or lithium disilicate ceramics. In the anterior sextant, the presence of more than 50% enamel substrate left (in the absence of any discoloration) favors the use of feldspathic porcelain owing to their high translucency and optical properties (**Fig. 5**). However, when the amount of enamel left is less than 50% or in the presence of discoloration, lithium disilicates are the material of choice (**Figs. 6–8**). In the posterior sextants feldspathic porcelains are contraindicated owing to their low mechanical properties. For lithium disilicate ceramic restoration, the clinician should always consider bonding to tooth structure of underlying substrate material. However, for alumina or zirconia restorations bonding is needed only if the retention is compromised (<3 mm height or a >20° convergence angel).

5. Translucency: To achieve successful esthetic outcomes, it is important to consider translucency versus opacity of the ceramic restorative material. Generally, in the esthetic zone, a high translucent material is desired, whereas for posterior region high opacity is more favorable (**Fig. 9**).

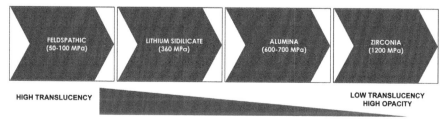

Fig. 9. Comparison of the mechanical and optical of discussed dental ceramics in the current review.

REFERENCES

1. da Silva LH, de Lima E, Miranda RBP, et al. Dental ceramics: a review of new materials and processing methods. Braz Oral Res 2017;31:133–46.
2. Bajraktarova-Valjakova E, Korunoska-Stevkovska V, Kapusevska B, et al. Contemporary dental ceramic materials, a review: chemical composition, physical and mechanical properties, indications for use. Open Access Maced J Med Sci 2018;6:1742–55.
3. Zarone F, Russo S, Sorrentino R. From porcelain-fused-to-metal to zirconia: clinical and experimental considerations. Dent Mater 2011;27:83–96.
4. Bajraktarova-Valjakova, Korunoska-Stevkovska, Kapusevska, et al. Contemporary Dental Ceramic Materials: Chemical Composition, Physical and Mechanical Properties. Open Access Macedonian Journal of Medical Sciences 2018;6(9): 1742–55.
5. Nikolopoulou F, Loukidis M, Proffesor A. Critical Review and evaluation of composite/ceramic onlays versus crowns. 2014. https://doi.org/10.4172/2157-7633. 1000261.
6. Edelhoff D, Brix O. All-ceramic restorations in different indications: a case series. J Am Dent Assoc 2011;142:14S–9S.
7. Kelly JR, Benetti P. Ceramic materials in dentistry: historical evolution and current practice. Aust Dent J 2011;56:84–96.
8. Gracis S, Thompson V, Ferencz J, et al. A new classification system for All-ceramic and ceramic-like restorative materials. Int J Prosthodont 2016;28: 227–35.
9. Shenoy A, Shenoy N. Dental ceramics: an update. J Conserv Dent 2010;13:195.
10. Saint-Jean SJ. Dental Glasses and Glass-ceramics. Adv. Ceram. Dent., Elsevier Inc.; 2014, p. 255–277. https://doi.org/10.1016/B978-0-12-394619-5.00012-2.
11. Montazerian M, Zanotto ED. Restorative dental glass-ceramics: current status and trends. Clin. Appl. Biomater. State-of-the-Art Progress, Trends, Nov. Approaches, Springer International Publishing; 2017, p. 313–336. https://doi.org/10.1007/978-3-319-56059-5_9.
12. Fu L, Engqvist H, Xia W. Glass–Ceramics in Dentistry: A Review. Materials 2020; 13(5):1049.
13. Ho GW, Matinlinna JP. Insights on Ceramics as Dental Materials. Part I: Ceramic Material Types in Dentistry. Silicon 2011;3:109–15.
14. Fu L, Xie L, Fu W, et al. Ultrastrong translucent glass ceramic with nanocrystalline, biomimetic structure. Nano Lett 2018;18:7146–54.
15. Montazerian M, Zanotto ED. Bioactive and inert dental glass-ceramics. J Biomed Mater Res A 2017;105:619–39.
16. Ritzberger C, Apel E, Höland W, et al. Properties and clinical application of three types of dental glass-ceramics and ceramics for CAD-CAM technologies. Materials (Basel) 2010;3:3700–13.
17. Lawson NC, Bansal R, Burgess JO. Wear, strength, modulus and hardness of CAD/CAM restorative materials. Dent Mater 2016;32(11):e275–83.
18. Hallmann L, Ulmer P, Gerngross MD, et al. Properties of hot-pressed lithium silicate glass-ceramics. Dent Mater 2019;35(5):713–29.
19. Mirmohammadi H. Resin-based ceramic matrix composite materials in dentistry. Adv. Ceram. Matrix Compos. Second Ed., Elsevier Inc.; 2018, p. 741–762. https://doi.org/10.1016/B978-0-08-102166-8.00030-X.
20. Code on Dental Procedures and Nomenclature (CDT) n.d. Available at: https://www.ada.org/en/publications/cdt. Accessed March 13, 2020.

21. Ben-Nissan B, Choi AH, Cordingley R. Alumina ceramics. Bioceram. their Clin. Appl., Elsevier Inc.; 2008, p. 223–242. https://doi.org/10.1533/9781845694227. 2.223.
22. Scherrer SS, Quinn GD, Quinn JB. Fractographic failure analysis of a Procera® AllCeram crown using stereo and scanning electron microscopy. Dent Mater 2008;24:1107–13.
23. Bona AD, Pecho OE, Alessandretti R. Zirconia as a dental biomaterial. Materials (Basel) 2015;8:4978–91.
24. Manziuc M-M, Gasparik C, Negucioiu M, et al. Optical properties of translucent zirconia: a review of the literature. EuroBiotech J 2019,3.45–51.
25. Gautam C, Joyner J, Gautam A, et al. Zirconia based dental ceramics: structure, mechanical properties, biocompatibility and applications. Dalton Trans 2016;45: 19194–215.

Adhesive Dentistry
Understanding the Science and Achieving Clinical Success

Marc Hayashi, DMD, MBA

KEYWORDS

- Adhesive • Dentin bonding agent • Acid-etch • Bond durability • Dentin sealing
- Postoperative sensitivity • Moist bonding • Solvent evaporation

KEY POINTS

- Understanding bonding agent classification helps to quickly clarify the benefits and drawbacks of adhesive groups, and explains the unique properties of universal adhesives.
- Enamel and dentin are very different substrates that require different approaches with adhesive application.
- Key steps in adhesive application include acid-etching, moist bonding, and solvent removal.
- Bond degradation occurs over time, but it can be lessened with the application of various agents to the cavity preparation.

INTRODUCTION

One of the most overlooked steps in adhesive dentistry is the application of the bonding agent. A proper understanding of the science behind these materials is of paramount importance in achieving consistent and predictable clinical outcomes. Unfortunately, this step in adhesive dentistry can be hard to teach objectively, and few dental schools or continuing education courses provide the opportunity to test parameters like bond strength on natural teeth. Practitioners thus become reliant on clinical outcomes and recollection of what they have learned in school. Furthermore, practitioners have numerous options to choose from, with each adhesive seemingly superior to others and each having varying application protocols.

It is worth noting that adhesives have undergone tremendous improvement over the years since their initial introduction in 1955 with Buonocore's[1] research on resin bonding to etched enamel surfaces, and later the introduction of bonding filling material to etched dentin by Fusayama and colleagues.[2] Advancements have favored simplicity, with subsequent reductions in the number of application steps down to

UCLA School of Dentistry, 10833 Le Conte Ave, Box 951668, Los Angeles, CA 90095, USA
E-mail address: mhayashi@dentistry.ucla.edu

Dent Clin N Am 64 (2020) 633–643
https://doi.org/10.1016/j.cden.2020.05.001
0011-8532/20/© 2020 Elsevier Inc. All rights reserved.

the single bottle materials widely used today. However, one must remember that simplicity does not always translate to improvement, and proper understanding of the material used is critical to achieving clinical success.

Adhesive Classification

The first step to improving clinical outcomes is knowing which bonding agent is being used. But to know that, one must understand that essentially all bonding agents are composed of 3 major components in some form, including an acid-etchant, primer, and adhesive. These components are separated or combined in various manners to create the adhesives available today. These combinations create the classification systems that help quickly distinguish one adhesive from another. Perhaps the easiest classification is by inclusion or separation of the acid-etch component. Bonding agents with a separate phosphoric acid etch step are termed "etch-and-rinse," whereas those with the acid-etch included in the adhesive are termed "self-etch." Within these categories themselves, the number of application steps varies. The manufacturer's instructions included with the adhesive will state the required application protocol, providing the practitioner with the information needed to assign a classification. A summary of the classification breakdown is seen in **Table 1**.

Classification Characteristics

Now that it has been determined which adhesive system is being used, one can begin to understand the pros and cons of each. For simplicity, each bonding agent will be referred to by its generation number going forward. At this juncture, it is also important to understand that the fifth and seventh generation bonding agents will tend to have similar characteristics, whereas the fourth and sixth generation bonding agents will have their own similar characteristics. The reason for this distinction is the presence of a neutral adhesive layer, which is provided by a separate step involving the adhesive alone.[3] This means that the acidic priming resin, characteristic of the fifth and seventh generation group, will be separated from the composite placed on top. This separation is key, allowing for the creation of a hydrophobic adhesive layer that is also more resistant to hydrolysis over time. This also allows fourth and sixth generation adhesives to be compatible with dual-cure and self-cure composites.[3] A summary of the characteristics of these bonding agent groups is listed in **Table 2**.

Given the benefits of the fourth and sixth generation adhesives, we would expect this to translate to clinical success. Interestingly, a systematic review by Peumans and colleagues[4] evaluated the effectiveness of contemporary adhesives placed in noncarious cervical lesion clinical trials between 1950 and 2013. It was found that

Table 1
Adhesive classification by total-etch/self-etch, number of steps, and generation

Classification	Steps	Generation	Examples
Etch-and-rinse	Etch, rinse, prime, bond (4 steps)	4th	OptiBond FL (Kerr); Scotchbond Multi-Purpose (3M)
Etch-and-rinse	Etch, rinse, prime + bond (3 steps)	5th	OptiBond Solo Plus (Kerr); Tenure Quik with Fluoride (DenMat)
Self-etch	Etch + prime, bond (2 steps)	6th	Clearfil SE Bond (Kuraray)
Self-etch	Etch + prime + bond (1 step)	7th	Prompt L-Pop (3M)

Table 2
Characteristics of bonding agent groups

Group	Pros	Cons
4th and 6th generation	• Neutral adhesive/hydrophobic layer separates acidic/hydrophilic primer from composite • Compatible with dual-cure and self-cure composites • More hydrolysis resistant bond	• Technique sensitivity during placement, especially with 4th generation
5th and 7th generation	• Less technique sensitivity with application • Reduced number of steps (7th generation)	• More acidic and hydrophilic • Some require dual-cure activator with self-cure/dual-cure composites or luting cements

the glass ionomers and two-step self-etch mild adhesives (2SEa-6th generation) displayed the most favorable and durable clinical bonding performance.[4] The 3-step etch-and-rinse adhesives (3E&Ra-4th generation) also performed favorably in this study, providing further evidence to support the use of these adhesives.

This study also highlighted an interesting finding in clinical effectiveness within the self-etch adhesives. If the pH of the adhesive was less than 1.5, it was termed strong, whereas a pH of greater than 1.5 was termed mild. When a strong pH adhesive was used, it was associated with a higher annual failure rate for self-etch adhesives. This conclusion is important, as it has implications in the discussion of the next group of adhesives, the universal bonding agents.

Universal Bonding Agents

Universal adhesives have gained in popularity due to their simplicity of use, versatility, and clinical effectiveness. The definition of a universal adhesive, however, is still vague, as the term "universal" seems to imply it can be used in all different ways at all times (self-etch, total-etch, self-cure, dual-cure, light-cure, bonds to tooth, bonds to composites, metals, ceramics, and zirconia), all while coming in one bottle. If that were the definition, it could be argued that no such adhesive currently exists. Nonetheless, it appears that these universal adhesives are here to stay and are deserving of a classification all their own.

One of the key benefits of universal adhesives is their ability to be used for both indirect and direct restorations. This means they can be used with direct composites, as well as bonding a veneer or crown. This versatility reduces the number of materials needed in the practice without compromising the quality of the restoration. What makes this versatility possible in many of the universal adhesives is the inclusion of the adhesive monomer 10 methacryloyloxydecyl-dihydrogen-phosphate (10-MDP for short). This monomer is the same one that has been used for many years in Kuraray's Panavia adhesive resin cement (Osaka, Japan). With its addition, the adhesive can bond to methacrylate-based restoratives and cements, as well as to tooth, metal and zirconia.[5] 10-MDP is also a highly hydrophobic monomer, making it less prone to water sorption and hydrolytic breakdown.[3] In addition, it can bond chemically to the tooth via its interaction with calcium in the hydroxyapatite of the tooth, forming stable MDP-Ca salts, which, along with nano-layering, explain the high stability of this bond and resistance to degradation.[6]

As stated previously, the pH of the adhesive seems to play an important role in clinical effectiveness, with a milder pH being beneficial. Although a mild pH self-etch adhesive is desired on dentin,[7] it is a concern on enamel, as the ability to adequately etch the substrate is in question. To improve this bond, the popular selective-etch technique is recommended.[7,8] This is where the enamel margin is etched with phosphoric acid, rinsed, dried, and then followed by placement of the universal adhesive. When used in this manner, a positive effect on the bond durability is noted.[9]

Another concern with pH of the adhesives is the effect of its compatibility with dual-cure and self-cure composites and resin cements.[8] In general, a stronger acidity/lower pH means less compatibility. Without proper polymerization at the adhesive interface, we have no bond. To overcome this, the use of dual-cure activators or amine-free cements must be used.[8] Thus, it is critical to read the manufacturer's instructions regarding the adhesive being used, as different adhesives have differing formulations. It should also be noted here that it is advised to not mix and match adhesives and resin cements when possible. With different chemistries present, adequate polymerization may not be occurring, thus negatively impacting the bond and clinical outcome.

ADHESIVE APPLICATION TECHNIQUE
Tooth Preparation

Before discussing the application technique of bonding agents, we need to go back a step further. Although seemingly insignificant, the bur used in the tooth and cavity preparation process is important. With the enamel being etched by phosphoric acid, we focus on the dentin. Although both carbide and diamond burs are used in the cavity preparation process, carbide burs are recommended on the dentin due to the thinner smear layer and higher bond strengths they create when using a self-etching adhesive.[10,11] When using an etch-and-rinse technique on dentin, no difference in bond strength was noted with respect to bur type used, although the bond strengths were all lower than the self-etch adhesive.[11]

Another factor to consider is the cavity preparation depth. Although enamel is relatively homogeneous throughout, dentin properties and composition vary considerably depending on the distance from the pulp. It has been shown that deeper dentin (closer to the pulp) exhibits lower bond strengths than superficial dentin (closer to the dentinoenamel junction), regardless of the adhesive system used.[12] This finding demonstrates the importance of intertubular dentin, which increases in total area toward the enamel. As the intertubular dentin increases, the dentinal tubule volume decreases, promoting greater development of the hybrid layer as coined by Nakabayashi and colleagues,[13] which appears to be more important for bond strength than resin tag development.[12] Furthermore, the deeper the dentin, the more permeable the substrate due to greater tubule diameter and number.[14] This increase in permeability can negatively influence the bond strength achieved at the adhesive interface,[15] especially for the etch-and-rinse adhesives in which the phosphoric acid removes the peritubular dentin and completely opens the tubules.[16] Thus, one proposed method of counteracting this fluid movement is through the use of local anesthetics with vasoconstrictors along with mild self-etching adhesives, which function to both decrease the pulpal pressure in the tooth and leave the smear plugs in the tubules largely intact, respectively.[17]

Adhesive Application

Regardless of the adhesive used, following the manufacturer's instructions is essential. Each will have slightly different protocols and recommended application times that are tailored to the specific chemistry of that adhesive. Nonetheless, a few key principles apply to all adhesives during the application process.

Acid-Etch Application

As mentioned previously, there is a general concern regarding the ability of self-etching adhesives being strong enough to adequately condition the enamel to the level of that achieved with 35% to 37% phosphoric acid, especially with uncut enamel. Thus, etching the enamel through the selective-etch technique is often advocated with self-etch adhesives,[7] as higher bond strengths have been reported when compared with enamel treated with the self-etch adhesives alone.[18] An application time of 15 seconds appears necessary to adequately condition the enamel surface, with longer etch times increasing surface roughness but producing no significant increase in bond strength.[18]

In the dentin, 15 seconds also appears adequate to achieving adequate bond strength, as longer etching times have been shown to reduce bond strength.[19] However, as is often the case in the clinical setting, we often run into nonideal dentin substrate. One such variation is that of sclerotic and older dentin, which has been shown to be more acid-resistant and require longer etching times in the range of 20 to 30 seconds.[20,21] Longer etching times however negatively affects any normal surrounding dentin, making subsequent adhesive infiltration more challenging.[21]

Moist Bonding

Contrary to enamel, in which we often look for the "frosty" appearance after rinsing and drying of the phosphoric acid, dentin is a very different substrate that behaves differently. After etching and rinsing, effort should be made to avoid overdrying the dentin. This is because of the collapse of the collagen matrix and decreased infiltration by the adhesive that results, producing decreased bond strengths, leakage, and sensitivity.[22] Dentin should thus remain moist during the application process. This is the reason for the often stated shiny or hydrated appearance to the surface that should be present after etching and rinsing.

Various methods can be used to achieve this appearance, including gentle air-drying, blot drying, or suction tip.[23,24] With the use of self-etch adhesives, the guesswork is largely removed, as no rinsing is involved. Interestingly, a study by Unlu and colleagues[25] compared self-etch and etch-and-rinse adhesives amongst dental providers with varied experience levels. They found that bond strengths achieved were higher with the self-etch method across all levels and that operator experience does influence the values obtained.

Solvent Removal

Proper evaporation of the solvent is perhaps one of the most overlooked steps in adhesive application. The solvent is water, ethanol, acetone, or some combination in the bonding agent. Water/ethanol-based solvents have been demonstrated to perform better than acetone-based solvents, largely due to the thinner adhesive layer generated.[26] Nonetheless, failure to evaporate the solvent has been shown to lead to poor bond strengths and nanoleakage as a result of dilution, incomplete polymerization, and phase separation of the adhesive. Consequently, longer air-drying times may be beneficial.[27] In addition, active agitation of the adhesive can help aid removal of the solvent through enhanced movement of monomer inward and solvent outward, thus improving the bond strength achieved and clinical performance.[28,29] To aid this step, the use of rigid microbrushes is recommended over flexible or long fiber-based ones in which adequate application pressure cannot be achieved.[29]

It is important that this principal of air thinning with solvents not be directly applied to the adhesive portion of the bonding agent. For instance, in fourth and sixth generation adhesives, in which the adhesive is applied in a separate step, caution should be exercised with excessive or prolonged air thinning, as this may significantly reduce the dentin bond strength. As a result, thinning the adhesive with a microbrush may be a superior alternative to air thinning.[30]

Bond Durability

It is known that the resin-dentin bonds decrease over time, and that this phenomenon is due to the degradation of the resin and collagen fibrils responsible for bond formation.[31] Matrix metalloproteinases (MMPs) have largely been implicated as the primary enzymes contributing to this degradation, which become activated during dentin bonding procedures.[32] Thus, to extend the life of this bond and improve its durability, several techniques are advocated. One such technique is to simply apply multiple coats of the adhesive.[29] Although there does not appear to be uniform agreement on the number of coats needed, doing so has been demonstrated to decrease the degradation rate with self-etch adhesives and improve the overall performance.[33]

Another technique with much interest is the use of an MMP inhibitor, with the most widely known agent being Chlorhexidine. Common agents using chlorhexidine include Cavity Cleanser (BISCO, Inc, Schaumberg, IL) and Consepsis (Ultradent, Inc, South Jordan, UT). Even at low concentrations, chlorhexidine has been shown to be effective in preventing degradation at the adhesive interface after acid-etching.[29] An application time of 15 to 30 seconds appears to be all that is necessary for effectiveness.[34] Use of chlorhexidine with self-etch adhesives on the other hand is not as conclusive. Although its placement on the dentin substrate before self-etch placement has shown some promise,[35] further research is necessary to validate this method.

Benzalkonium chloride is another agent that has demonstrated MMP inhibition properties.[36] This agent is included in the acid etchants of BISCO Inc and is included in the cavity disinfectant Tubulicid Red (Dental Therapeutics, Saltsjo-Boo, Sweden), and has been shown to strongly bind to demineralized dentin even after rinsing.[36] When compared with untreated teeth showing decreases in bond strength after 6 and 12 months, the use of benzalkonium chloride demonstrated stable bond strengths over the same period.[37] In addition, glutaraldehyde containing desensitizers such as Gluma (Kulzer, Hanau, Germany) have been implicated as MMP inhibitors in matrix-bound dentin, contributing to prevention of collagen degradation.[38] However, it's impact on bond strength of overlying resin remains unclear, with conflicting evidence available.[39,40] It should also be noted that this agent is marketed primarily for desensitizing reasons, and has cytotoxicity concerns.[41,42] Thus, its use on acid-etched dentin remains unclear at present and warrants additional investigation.

Light Curing

Once the adhesive is placed, light curing is generally required among most bonding agents to maximize the bond strength achieved. This critical step can easily be overlooked, as it often receives less attention than most other topics. Nevertheless, proper knowledge and technique with curing lights is of paramount importance in the dental practice, as it allows the provider to provide much of today's dental procedures, from sealants and composites to bonded indirect restorations. It is no surprise then that its correct use is critical to the successful execution of adhesive dentistry.

It should be kept in mind, however, that high-power light-emitting diode curing lights available today are able to generate significant increases in temperature.[43] This is especially important when curing the bonding agent in deep preparations where little dentin remains over the pulp, as pulpal damage can occur.[44] Although increasing the distance from the curing light to the dentin may decrease the temperature, compromised polymerization may result, especially in areas difficulty for the light to reach.[43] One method that shows promise to reduce the temperature rise with prolonged light curing is directing a stream of air at the tooth during light exposure.[45] In addition, undercuts may be present in the cavity preparation, producing shadows and areas of poor light exposure. This may require the operator to move the curing light around over a longer period of time to ensure polymerization of all areas.[43]

In any case, it is important that this critical step be carried out correctly to ensure adequate polymerization of the light cured adhesive and resins. In addition to technique, simple steps that can be taken to optimize the output from the curing light include periodic monitoring with a radiometer and routine examination of the light tip for damage and debris.[43] Clear barrier sleeves and wraps can also be used as a method of protection for the light tip during treatment to minimize contamination without significantly compromising the curing of resin or the light spectrum emitted.[46]

IMMEDIATE VERSUS DELAYED DENTIN SEALING

Immediate dentin sealing (IDS) is the application of an adhesive to freshly cut dentin after preparation for an indirect restoration, such as an onlay or crown, and before the final impression.[3] This allows for pre-polymerization of the adhesive and stress-free dentin bond development, as well as protection from bacterial leakage and sensitivity during the provisional phase.[47] This differs from delayed dentin sealing (DDS) in which the adhesive is placed right before seating of the restoration but is left unpolymerized. A study by Magne and colleagues[47] demonstrated that the bond strength achieved through the IDS protocol resulted in a significant increase in bond strength over the DDS technique and reduces concern regarding incomplete seating. The IDS technique also calls for the use of a filled adhesive, such as the fourth generation OptiBond FL (Kerr, Orange, CA). Such an adhesive develops a uniform layer that is, thick enough to resist subsequent re-exposure of dentin during cleaning and preparation procedures that occur before final indirect restoration seating.[48]

Although this technique appears effective, it can be technique sensitive, as resin based provisionals can stick to the adhesive during fabrication, making retrieval difficult.[47,48] A thick layer of petroleum jelly or another separating medium is thus necessary to prevent this bond from occurring.[47] In addition, polyether-based impression material cannot be used with this technique, as faulty impressions have been shown to occur over 50% of the time due to impression material adhering to the adhesive surface. This phenomenon did not occur with air blocking and pumicing of the adhesive with a vinyl polysiloxane material.[49]

POSTOPERATIVE SENSITIVITY

Postoperative sensitivity is a longstanding and common clinical problem that dentists encounter with adhesive dentistry.[50] Many efforts have been made to reduce its incidence as outlined previously. From an adhesive standpoint, self-etch adhesives have a purported benefit of less postoperative sensitivity given their incomplete removal of the smear layer, with tubules remaining partially plugged.[7] Nonetheless, the difference in postoperative sensitivity between etch-and-rinse and self-etch adhesives appears to be minimal,[51,52] with operator technique being more influential than the type of adhesive used.[51]

Another commonly held belief is the use of a glass-ionomer lining material under the resin composite restoration to minimize the incidence of postoperative sensitivity.

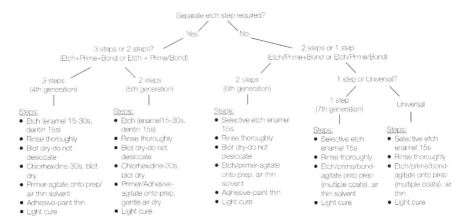

Fig. 1. Understanding your adhesive.

However, a study by Burrow examined this technique, and found no difference in post-operative sensitivity between restorations placed with or without a glass-ionomer liner, regardless of the bonding agent used (total-etch or self-etch).[53] Furthermore, Blum and Wilson[54] demonstrated that the available evidence does not support the routine placement of liners, unless it is intended to have a therapeutic effect.

UNDERSTANDING YOUR ADHESIVE

With the preceding information in hand, we can now apply the principles to our adhesives used in daily practice. **Fig. 1** provides a decision tree to help understand which adhesive is being used, and the steps that are generally required in its application. It is critical to remember that all products may have slight differences in application times based on their chemistries, and that following the instructions for use is of the utmost importance.

SUMMARY

Adhesive dentistry has undoubtedly experienced tremendous improvements since Buonocore's[1] initial introduction of enamel etching in the 1950s. Although the improvements have been significant and largely intended to reduce technique sensitivity and the number of steps, certain key principles remain the same. Given certain limitations with several adhesives, as outlined previously, the practitioner may even want to consider using a couple of different adhesives for various situations. Regardless of the approach, it should be reemphasized that careful application technique and attention to detail during adhesive placement, along with following the manufacturer's instructions, are key considerations in the pursuit of delivering quality and long-lasting adhesive dental care.

REFERENCES

1. Buonocore MG. A simple method of increasing the adhesion of acrylic filling materials to enamel surfaces. J Dent Res 1955;34(6):849–53.
2. Fusayama T, Nakamura M, Kurosaki N, et al. Non-pressure adhesion of a new adhesive restorative resin. J Dent Res 1979;58(4):1364–70.
3. Suh BI. Principles of adhesion dentistry: a theoretical and clinical guide for dentists. Newton (PA): Aegis Publications LLC; 2013. p. 11–57, 119-138.

4. Peumans M, De Munck JD, Mine A, et al. Clinical effectiveness of contemporary adhesives for the restoration of non-carious cervical lesions. A systematic review. Dent Mater 2014;30:1089–103.
5. Alex G. Universal adhesives: the next evolution in adhesive dentistry? Compend Contin Educ Dent 2015;36(1):15–26.
6. Yoshida Y, Yoshihara K, Nagaoka N, et al. Self-assembled nano-layering at the adhesive interface. J Dent Res 2012;91(4):376–81.
7. Van Meerbeek B, Yoshihara K, Yoshida Y, et al. State of the art of self-etch adhesives. Dent Mater 2011;27:17–28.
8. Suh BI. Universal adhesives: The evolution of adhesive solutions continues. Compend Contin Educ Dent 2014;35(4):278.
9. Suzuki T, Takammizawa T, Barkmeier WW, et al. Influence of etching mode on enamel bond durability of universal adhesive systems. Oper Dent 2016;41(5):520–30.
10. Ogata M, Harada N, Yamaguchi S, et al. Effects of different burs on dentin bond strengths of self-etching primer bonding systems. Oper Dent 2001;26:375–82.
11. Oliveira SSA, Pugach MK, Hilton JF, et al. The influence of the dentin smear layer on adhesion: a self-etching primer vs. a total-etch system. Dent Mater 2003;19:758–67.
12. Sattabanasuk V, Shimada Y, Tagami J. The bond of resin to different dentin surface characteristics. Oper Dent 2004;29(3):333–41.
13. Nakabayashi N, Nakamura M, Yasuda N. Hybrid layer as a dentin-bonding mechanism. J Esthet Restor Dent 1991;3(4):133–8.
14. Garberoglio R, Brannstrom M. Scanning electron microscopic investigation of human dentinal tubules. Arch Oral Biol 1976;23:355–62.
15. Pashley DH, Carvalho RM. Dentine permeability and dentine adhesion. J Dent 1997;25:355–72.
16. Rosales-Leal JI, do la Torre-Moreno FJ, Bravo M. Effect of pulp pressure on the micropermeability and sealing ability of etch and rinse and self-etching adhesives. Oper Dent 2007;32(3):242–50.
17. Hebling J, Castro FLA, Costa CAS. Adhesive performance of dentin bonding agents applied in vivo and in vitro. Effect of intrapulpal pressure and dentin depth. J Biomed Mater Res B Appl Biomater 2007;83B:295–303.
18. Barkmeier WW, Erickson RL, Kimmes NS, et al. Effect of enamel etching time on roughness and bond strength. Oper Dent 2009;34(2):217–22.
19. Hashimoto M, Ohno H, Kaga M, et al. Over-etching effects on micro-tensile bond strength and failure patterns for two dentin bonding systems. J Dent 2002;30:99–105.
20. Lopes GC, Vieira LC, Araujo E, et al. Effect of dentin age and acid etching time on dentin bonding. J Adhes Dent 2011;13:139–45.
21. Prati C, Chersoni S, Mongiorgi R, et al. Thickness and morphology of resin-infiltrated dentin layer in young, old, and sclerotic dentin. Oper Dent 1999;24:66–72.
22. Pashley DH, Tay FR, Carvalho RM, et al. From dry bonding to water-wet bonding to ethanol-wet bonding. A review of the interactions between dentin matrix and solvated resins using a micromodel of the hybrid layer. Am J Dent 2007;20:7–21.
23. Magne P, Mahallati R, Bazos P, et al. Direct dentin bonding technique sensitivity when using air/suction drying steps. J Esthet Restor Dent 2008;20(2):130–8.
24. Nagpal R, Tewari S, Gupta R. Effect of various surface treatments on the microleakage and ultrastructure of resin-tooth interface. Oper Dent 2007;32(1):16–23.

25. Unlu N, Gunal S, Ulker M, et al. Influence of operator experience on in vitro bond strength of dentin adhesives. J Adhes Dent 2012;14:223–7.
26. Zander-Grande C, Ferreira SQ, da Costa TRF, et al. Application of etch-and-rinse adhesives on dry and rewet dentin under rubbing action: a 24-month clinical evaluation. J Am Dent Assoc 2011;142(7):828–35.
27. Hashimoto M, Tay FR, Svizero NR, et al. The effects of common errors on sealing ability of total-etch adhesives. Dent Mater 2006;22:560–8.
28. Reis A, Pellizzaro A, Dal-Bianco K, et al. Impact of adhesive application to wet and dry dentin on long-term resin-dentin bond strengths. Oper Dent 2007; 32(4):380–7.
29. Reis A, Carrilho M, Breschi L, et al. Overview of clinical alternatives to minimize the degradation of the resin-dentin bonds. Oper Dent 2013;38(4):E103–27.
30. Hilton TJ, Schwarts RS. The effect of air thinning on dentin adhesive bond strength. Oper Dent 1995;20:133–7.
31. Hashimoto M. A review-micromorphological evidence of degradation in resin-dentin bonds and potential preventional solutions. J Biomed Mater Res B Appl Biomater 2010;92B:268–80.
32. Tjaderhane L, Nascimento FD, Breschi L, et al. Optimizing dentin bond durability: control of collagen degradation my matrix metalloproteinases and cysteine cathepsins. Dent Mater 2013;29:116–35.
33. Ito S, Tay FR, Hashimoto M, et al. Effects of multiple coatings of two all-in-one adhesives on dentin bonding. J Adhes Dent 2005;7(2):133–41.
34. Loguercio AD, Stanislawczuk R, Polli LG, et al. Influence of chlorhexidine digluconate concentration and application time on resin-dentin bond strength durability. Eur J Oral Sci 2009;117:587–96.
35. Campos EA, Correr GM, Leonardi DP, et al. Chlorhexidine diminishes the loss of bond strength over time under simulated pulpal pressure and thermo-mechanical stressing. J Dent 2009;37(2):108–14.
36. Tezvergil-Mutluay A, Mutluay MM, Gu L, et al. The anti-MMP activity of benzalkonium chloride. J Dent 2011;39(1):57–64.
37. Sabatini C, Pashley DH. Aging of adhesive interfaces treated with benzalkonium chloride and benzalkonium methacrylate. Eur J Oral Sci 2015;123(2):102–7.
38. Sabatini C, Scheffel DLS, Scheffel RH, et al. Inhibition of endogenous human dentin MMPs by Gluma. Dent Mater 2014;30(7):752–8.
39. Huh JB, Kim JH, Chung MK, et al. The effect of several dentin desensitizers on shear bond strength of adhesive resin luting cement using self-etching primer. J Dent 2008;36(12):1025–32.
40. Stawarczyk B, Hartmann L, Hartmann R, et al. Impact of gluma desensitizer on the tensile strength of zirconia crowns bonded to dentin: an in vitro study. Clin Oral Investig 2012;16:201–13.
41. Eyuboglu GB, Yesilyurt C, Erturk M. Evaluation of cytotoxicity of dentin desensitizing products. Oper Dent 2015;40(5):503–14.
42. Lee J, Sabatini C. Glutaraldehyde collagen cross-linking stabilizes resin-dentin interfaces and reduces bond degradation. Eur J Oral Sci 2017;125:63–71.
43. Price RBT. Light curing in dentistry. Dent Clin North Am 2017;61:751–78.
44. Mouhat M, Mercer J, Stangvaltaite L, et al. Light-curing units used in dentistry: factors associated with heat development-potential risk for patients. Clin Oral Investig 2017;21:1687–96.
45. Rueggeberg FA, Giannini M, Arrais CAG, et al. Light curing in dentistry and clinical implications: a literature review. Braz Oral Res 2017;31(suppl):64–91.

46. Scott BA, Felix CA, Price RBT. Effect of disposable infection control barriers on light output from dental curing lights. J Can Dent Assoc 2004;70(2):105–10.
47. Magne P, Kim TH, Cascione D, et al. Immediate dentin sealing improves bond strength of indirect restorations. J Prosthet Dent 2005;94:511–9.
48. Magne P. Immediate dentin sealing: a fundamental procedure for indirect bonded restorations. J Esthet Restor Dent 2005;17:144–55.
49. Magne P, Nielsen B. Interactions between impression materials and immediate dentin sealing. J Prosthet Dent 2009;102(5):298–305.
50. Christensen GJ. Preventing postoperative tooth sensitivity in class I, II and V restorations. J Am Dent Assoc 2002;133:229–31.
51. Perdigao J, Geraldeli S, Hodges JS. Total-etch versus self-etch adhesive: effect on postoperative sensitivity. J Am Dent Assoc 2003;134(2):1621–9.
52. Scotti N, Bergantin E, Giovannini R, et al. Influence of multi-step etch-and-rinse versus self-etch adhesive systems on the post-operative sensitivity in medium-depth carious lesions: an in vivo study. Am J Dent 2015;28:214–8.
53. Burrow MF, Banomyong D, Harnirattisai C, et al. Effect of glass-ionomer cement lining on postoperative sensitivity in occlusal cavities restored with resin composite-a randomized clinical trial. Oper Dent 2009;34(6):648–55.
54. Blum IR, Wilson NHF. An end to linings under posterior composites? J Am Dent Assoc 2018;149(3):209–13.

Implementing Digital Dentistry into Your Esthetic Dental Practice

Lawrence Fung, DDS[a],*, Phil Brisebois, BA[b]

KEYWORDS

- Digital dentistry • Intra oral scanners • Smile design • CAD/CAM milling
- 3D printing

KEY POINTS

- The use of digital dentistry is on the increase as costs to acquire digital technology have gone down dramatically and allowed for more practitioners to integrate digital equipment with reduced investment.
- One of the most significant benefits of digital technology in dentistry is the ability to streamline processes that can be cumbersome via the analog way.
- In digital dentistry, it is important to understand the advantages and disadvantages of each device or system available.

INTRODUCTION

When we look around, it is amazing yet eerie to see how surrounded we are by technology. The word *technology* comes from 2 Greek words, translated into *techne* and *logos*. *Techne* means art, skill, craft, or the way, manner, or means by which a thing is gained. *Logos* means word, the utterance by which inward thought is expressed, a saying, or an expression. Literally, then, technology means words or discourse about the way things are gained. In today's more relevant definition of technology, it can be broken down into 4 working subsets: technology, an object, knowledge, and last, a process. For the purposes of this article, the authors expand on all of these subsets for digital dentistry. Digital dentistry and its implementation into practice is more than just the piece of equipment. It is important to understand more than how to use the device, the nuances of the technology, the processes involved, and how the technology fits into your existing practice system.

[a] UCLA Center for Esthetic Dentistry Lecturer, 6101 West Centinela Avenue, Suite 375, Culver City, CA 90230, USA; [b] UCLA Center for Esthetic Dentistry Lecturer, Founder NOVO Dental Studios & GRAVIDEE, 465 N Roxbury, Suite 703, Beverly Hills, CA 90210, USA
* Corresponding author.
E-mail address: Lawrencf@ucla.edu

Dent Clin N Am 64 (2020) 645–657
https://doi.org/10.1016/j.cden.2020.07.003
0011-8532/20/© 2020 Elsevier Inc. All rights reserved.

As with anything new to an existing system, there are pros and cons of modifying a single process within the current work flow; digital applications are just additional tools in your toolbox, like a hammer and a screwdriver.

In digital dentistry, it is important to understand the advantages and disadvantages of each device or system available. From a well-rounded understanding, you will be able to see how and if it fits within your practice. Just like any other instrument, digital technology also has its limitations; in some situations digital technology works very well, whereas in other circumstances, digital technology may be contraindicated, similarly to using a screwdriver instead of a hammer. Herein, the authors discuss digital technology in dentistry, its advantages, shortcomings, and it potential to elevate how to practice contemporary dentistry with a vision to the future.

The use of digital dentistry is on the increase as costs to acquire digital technology (digital radiology, for example) have decreased dramatically and allowed for more practitioners to integrate digital equipment with reduced investment. For the purposes of this article, the authors focus on the acquisition of patient data by exploring digital intraoral scanners and digital radiography and they touch briefly on digital photography. They also look at the applications one can have with the digital data, and their potential outputs-associated 3-dimensional (3D) printing and milled restorations.

One of the most significant benefits of digital technology in dentistry is the ability to streamline processes that can be cumbersome via the analog way. The biggest incentive about creating more efficiency in a dental practice is the ability to provide consistent high-quality dentistry while decreasing costs for the patient. In any business, the net operating income, namely, the amount of money left over after expenses, is something that cannot be ignored, and therefore, reducing the chair time needed per procedure will bring about more revenue generated on a daily basis, and digital dentistry can speed up certain processes, allowing for a more efficiently run practice. In the authors' practice, for example, new patient data acquisition time was reduced dramatically with the use of digital technology, especially when considering the time needed for preliminary physical impressions, to pour up the models, to mount the case as well as to store the cases.

In the authors' practice, the new patient record includes a full set of photographs, intraoral scan, and a full-mouth radiograph set. A scan will allow the practitioner to evaluate the dentition and discuss with the patient immediately on a 3D model versus having to wait to pour up a case, mount on an articulator, and then bring the patient back to discuss the findings. Because data are stored digitally, the practitioner can reference the acquired data at any time, thus enabling the practitioner to go back into these digital files to reexamine the patient to ensure nothing was overlooked.

Another advantage of digital dentistry is how the practice can expand their boundaries when assembling the dental team. In an esthetic dental practice, having an exceptionally capable ceramist in the team and using digital technology enable the practitioner to work remotely and send patients' cases to practically any ceramist throughout the globe. In addition, with the quality of digital photography and its accuracy at capturing color, shade match can be done remotely as well. With the use of calibrated gray cards and polarized lens photography, accurate color information can be transmitted to the ceramist; this can eliminate the need for a custom shade appointment that would have normally had to be done in person by the ceramist.

Another noteworthy advantage of transitioning and embracing digital capabilities is demonstrating to existing as well as new patients how updated your approach is. Not only do patients appreciate seeing that their caregiver is up-to-date but also many admire clinicians who are leaders in technology, and they become your biggest advocates. By the same token, as patients become increasingly aware of advances in dentistry, if you do not have the updated technology in your office, they may question your professional abilities. One great example is with the significant advertising being done by those clear aligner therapy startups, such as Smile Direct Club, and how their stores feature intraoral scanners. As more and more of the public are aware of these scanning technologies, the more they expect it to be the norm.

DRAWBACKS OF DIGITAL TECHNOLOGY IN DENTISTRY?
Startup Costs

The costs are still relatively high when considering acquiring digital dental equipment. Many of the systems operate on a subscription-based licensing platform. For example, some Digital Smile Design Apps require a yearly subscription. Likewise, some intraoral scanners have a monthly or annual fee, and cloud-based data storage for backups often comes with a fee. Training is usually provided by the equipment distributor, but any advanced instructional use of technology is not. Because of the limited resources provided by many digital companies, the learning curve can be quite steep initially.

Lack of Standardized Work Flows

It is the authors' experience that digital dentistry currently lacks well-defined universal work flows that can be seamlessly integrated into any practice. Interoperability is an issue, and different data acquisition devices from different companies will export different file types. Although the universally accepted digital scan file is stereolithography (STL), some of the scanners will prefer to export in their own native scan files, such as a polygon file format (PLY) or in the case of 3shape, it will export as a Digital Imaging and Communications in Medicine format (DCM), which will need to be converted to STL.

Limited Access to Digital Partners

One of the biggest challenges of digital is finding other members of the dental team that use digital technology, because many of the higher-end small-scale laboratories are still not fully digital because of the lack of digital case submission volume. The cost for the small laboratories to acquire printing technology in-house and digital design software may not be economically feasible if most of their current client list is not digital.

Intraoral Scanners and Scanning

The following are some of the current popular scanners. In the graph, the pros and cons of each system are displayed. Speed and cost can vary, and there is no consistent correlation between those mentioned above and output quality. Some require additional equipment to operate them (like a laptop for 3Shape). Although some scanners may be more accurate, the size of the intraoral camera may be an obstacle for some circumstances, like capturing distobuccal cusp of maxillary second molars or a limited size oral cavity (ie, pediatric dentists and orthodontists). A learning curve and adjustment for scanning, and scanning sequence and digital workflow present other challenges when integrating digital impressions.[1] Also, determining deep marginal finish lines of prepared teeth[2] can be exceedingly more challenging and require an additional skill set to be learned.

The Digital Dentistry as part of the restorative process can be broken down into 3 step: Data-acquisition, design, and manufacturing. In this section, the different options and systems for digital impressions are discussed. Although there are several different digital impression systems on the market today, there are only 3 categories these systems can be categorized into: (1) scan only (stand alone); (2) scan, design, and output to a third-party mill; and (3) all-in-one ecosystem.

Stand-alone systems

There are several stand-alone systems on the market today; however, the following 5 would be considered the most relevant scanners. They include Cerec Primescan, Carestream CS, iMedit 500, iTero, and Trios. Each of these scanners makes a very high-quality digital impression, and all have specific features and benefits designed to enhance the user experience.

It is important to note that although each of these scanners will make an impression in color, that this color image is not always transferred to the laboratory for fabrication. In order to achieve the highest-quality restorative outcome, it is extremely important to understand the technology and software that your laboratory is using to process your digital impressions. For example, although itero, Carestream, Cerec, and Medit all make digital impressions in color, the STL that is provided to the laboratory for fabrication is a black and gray scale image, making it more challenging and most times impossible to mark the margin, especially with veneer and equigingival preparations.

Scan, design, and output to a third-party mill

The next category of products is used for scanning the patient, but also has the ability to add chair-side design software. Although purchased separately, Trios by 3Shape allows seamless integration, and with additional modules can be purchased directly from 3Shape and added to the Chairside Dental Desktop software. These modules include Implant Studio, Smile Design, Restorative Design, Ortho Simulator, Caries Detection, and the CAM software required to output design to an in-house mill. Other intraoral scanners can also be integrated as part of chair-side systems, but unlike 3Shape, use a second party design software called exocad ChairsideCAD.

All-in-One ecosystem

The systems available in this category are Planmeca Emerald and Sirona Cerec. These systems allow a dentist and team to make a digital impression of a patient in their office, use the internal design software to design a restoration for the patient, and mill that restoration using an integrated in-office mill. These systems have proven to be very successful for some users but require a very specific workflow to be clinically successful. Both systems are simple in their setup: included is an intraoral scanner with built-in design software and a mill with built in CAM software,"call it plug and play." The challenge lies in the processing of the material and patient timing. The 2 most commonly used materials in dentistry are Emax and zirconia, and both require post-processing and sintering times that range from 45 minutes to 10 hours. A true benefit can be seen using this technology to mill composite and polymethyl methacrylate for inlays/onlays and also temporaries. In addition, both the Planmeca Emerald and Sirona Cerec are also available as a stand-alone system, whereby digital impressions can be made and sent to the laboratory for fabrication.

When investing in technology, it is important to consider one's potential future use. If the goal is to eventually have the ability to be self-sufficient and produce most restorations in-office, it is important to consider the workflow and available options for each specific scanner system when planning a purchase. The integration and workflow are not as seamless as many manufacturers promote, and each system has their own nuances.

Just like the system setup for the dental operatory, the dental laboratory has a variety of different hardware and software that can be used to design and fabricate indirect fixed restorations, digital dentures, implant planning, surgical guides, and restorations, as well as other dental devices. Nowadays, most if not all dental prosthetics can be fabricated using CAD/CAM technology.

Although all systems are open and produce an STL file, the file format is in gray scale and does not demonstrate colors and therefore cannot differentiate between tooth and tissue colors. It is the responsibility of the scanner manufacturer to produce a color-ready file or alternatively a file that can export the finish-line position ready to be used by the laboratory for margin evaluation and restoration design. The inability to view the file in color may create a real challenge for the restorative dentist when evaluating a digital impression for finish-line reproducibility.

Regardless of the scanner's ability to import and export into laboratory software in color, they all work well to make digital impressions for crown and bridge, implants workflow, dental appliances, smile design, and treatment planning. The key with all of the systems still boils down to the quality of dentistry. None of the scanners have the ability to see through tissue, and therefore, it is essential that tissue be retracted properly from the margin, as well as preventing fluids from hindering a qualifying impression. Equally important, the digital impression must be evaluated on screen before being sent to the laboratory for fabrication (**Fig. 1**).

Fig. 2 demonstrates a workflow for the initial new patient visit. Once the data are acquired from the patient, the information is uploaded into the patient management software or onto a HIPPA-compliant storage program. With the use of digitally collected patient dental conditions, they can be viewed with the patient for clear communication and dental education.

The work flow chart in **Fig. 3** is for indirect restorations and or dental appliances, such as an occlusal guard. The process is not really different from the analog way; instead of making an impression with polyvinyl siloxane impression material, you would just capture the prepared data or dentition digitally. The biggest caveat of digital dentistry is the ability to have the preparation or impression sent to the laboratory immediately, saving pickup travel time, with zero risk for cross-contamination. Another big advantage of digital is the ability to review the preparation or impression to ensure there are no inaccuracies present that may warrant a new impression. A big advantage of digital for indirect preparations, especially onlay preparations, is the ability to see interocclusal reduction in real time to help reduce underreduction. Reviewing preparations in real time in occlusion will also help aid the practitioner from overreducing preparations as well, allowing for the esthetic dentist to be as minimally invasive as possible.

It is important to understand dental technology is changing at the fastest rate yet, and it is imperative to keep up-to-date. Luckily, there are more resources available online than ever, including continuing education courses and forums that can easily be

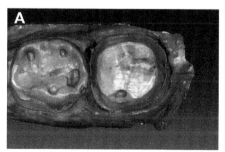
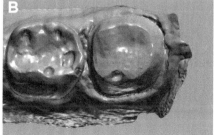

Fig. 1. (*A*) Scan made in color; (*B*) scan exported as a black and white STL into 3D software.

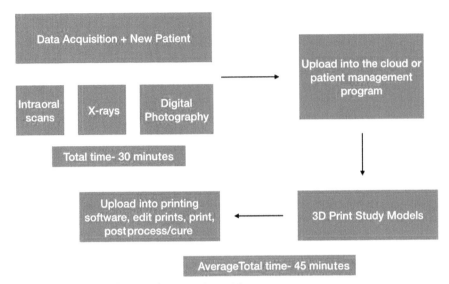

Fig. 2. Workflow for the initial new patient visit.

found on social media platforms that allow for crowdsourcing to help solve any digital dentistry problems the clinician may have.

DIGITAL WORKING PROTOTYPE

Fig. 4 is the result of performing a digital smile design from an intraoral mockup to a final product. Doing a digital wax-up is a great way for patients to preview and try out their final product without any kind of tooth preparation.

The initial presentation of the patient was the top image. The chief complaint was that the patient did not like the diastema between #8 and #9 and that the laterals felt too narrow. The patient also had some bonding done before but was tired of the need to keep replacing the composites and wanted something more long term. With digital smile design, we were able to show the patient a visual representation of the proposed changes. Once the patient approved the digital smile design, an intraoral mockup was done to verify fit, esthetics, and phonetics of the new proposed restorations. Once the patient signed off on the intraoral mockup, the scan was sent to

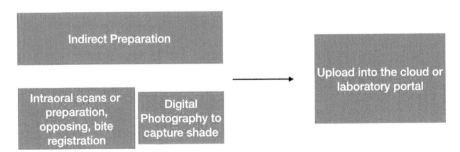

Fig. 3. Workflow for indirect restorations and or dental appliances, such as an occlusal guard.

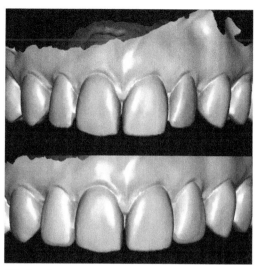

Fig. 4. Digitally modified smile.

the orthodontist, and they used it as a guide to close the diastema between #8 and #9 and create some restorative spacing on the mesial and distal of #7 and #10 to allow for minimal reduction for the proposed feldspathic veneers.

A summary of the whole procedure as seen in **Fig. 5** is from start to final product. The case was done digitally and remotely with a laboratory, and shade matching was only done chair-side with photography; no try-in was needed. The patient did not have to travel to the laboratory, saving time and allowing for the practice and patient to use any ceramist in the world.

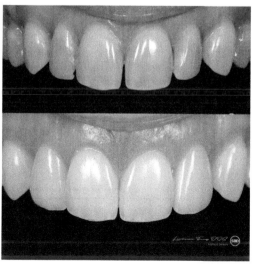

Fig. 5. Initial and postrestorations and orthodontics. (*Courtesy of* Lawrence Fung, DDS, Culver City, CA.)

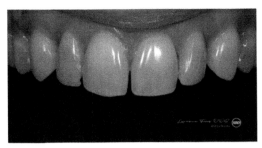

Fig. 6. Initial presentation. (*Courtesy of* Lawrence Fung, DDS, Culver City, CA.)

The chief complaint is the narrow laterals that were restored with conservative composite restorations and the diastema between the 2 centrals (**Fig. 6**). The patient not only wanted to close the diastema between the centrals but also wanted more fuller-looking lateral incisors. The patient wanted the least minimally invasive procedure done.

In this case, once the digital wax-up was provided by the digital designer, using a SprintRay Pro (Los Angeles, California), the models for putty matrix fabrication and evaluation were printed in-house (**Fig. 7**). The SprintRay Pro (**Figs. 8** and **9**) is a digital light projector (DLP) printer that can print 2 inches in height per hour, so in this case, the print took about 45 minutes. For 3D printing, there are DLP and SLA (STL). The latter is significantly older but more accurate yet slower than the former. DLP, however, is starting to catch up in micron accuracy. A big benefit of DLP is the machines are much less expensive than the SLA machines.[3] The SprintRay Pro, which was used to print the smile design models, is a DLP.

The patient, after reviewing the smile preview, was able to have an intraoral mockup done to visualize immediately the proposed changes. Although the patient is wearing this mockup, the mockup can be adjusted intraorally, and the new contours can be scanned to help aid the digital designer when finessing the digital wax-up (**Fig. 10**). The digital wax-up will serve as a blueprint for the new final restorations and temporaries. The materials used for the intraoral mockup was Telio CS from Ivoclar. The putty matrix used to duplicate the wax-up to the dentition was Flexitime from Kulzer.

Fig. 11 shows 2 shades, one for the closest match and a second to offer as a comparison. The shade guide the author likes to use is VITA Classical. One of the biggest advantages of digital dentistry is increased efficiency in the workflow.

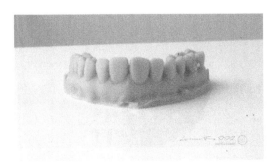

Fig. 7. Printed model. (*Courtesy of* Lawrence Fung, DDS, Culver City, CA.)

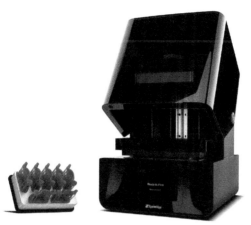

Fig. 8. SprintRay Pro 3D printer. (*Courtesy of* SprintRay, Los Angeles, CA.)

In **Fig. 12**, the shade identification is marked so the ceramist can verify the shade classification. Always include comparison shades as a way for the ceramist to calibrate color.

The filter removes unwanted reflections from the teeth that are caused by a flash. These highlights can send false information to the ceramist. In the cross-polarized photograph, you can see the hypersaturation of color and contrast much better (**Fig. 13**). These filters are great, especially where any decalcification may be present, and aids the ceramist when fabricating the custom restorations. The product the author uses is polar_eyes from PhotoMed.

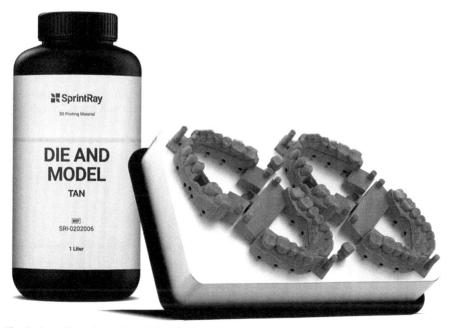

Fig. 9. SprintRay die and model resin. (*Courtesy* of SprintRay, Los Angeles, CA.)

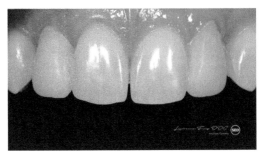

Fig. 10. Try-in of the digital smile preview. (*Courtesy of* Lawrence Fung, DDS, Culver City, CA.)

Once patient data are collected by the doctor and sent to the laboratory for fabrication, the design workflow becomes the same. When a dentist sends an impression to the laboratory, whether it is digital or conventional, the same process for designing and manufacturing will occur. A digital impression should be kept in a full digital workflow throughout the production process in order to eliminate inaccuracies.

Using digital technology allows the technician to evaluate the restoration preproduction while looking at all aspects of the case, including interocclusal spacing, emergence profile, margin position, and virtual articulator movements to evaluate restorations in function. The programs can then help the technician evaluate material requirements and help to determine if adequate space has been provided to produce the prescribed restoration. The system can also suggest different materials to produce a more subtle solution if preparations are less than ideal. The system and its precise calibration with manufacturer material specifications will also ensure consistent restorations will be fabricated.

With implants, digital technology allows for an easy transfer of information for transmucosal profile by simple scanning of the restorative site. **Fig. 14** is an example of a surgical plan with an immediate custom healing abutment that was designed from the preplanned implant coordinates, allowing the surgeon, restoring doctor, and laboratory to plan the most ideal position of the implant based on the desired prosthetic outcome. It also allows for the development of soft tissue from the time of implant placement. The custom healing abutment will begin to support

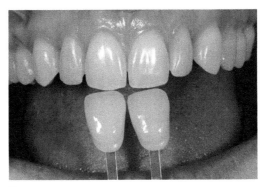

Fig. 11. Shade selection.

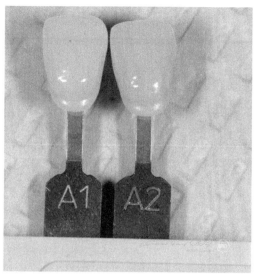

Fig. 12. Shade tabs chosen. (*Courtesy of* Lawrence Fung, DDS, Culver City, CA.)

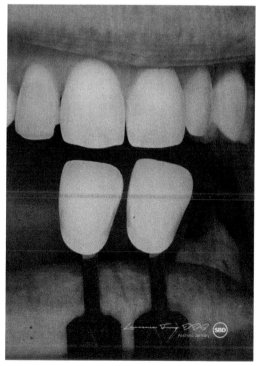

Fig. 13. Shade taken with cross-polarizing lens. (*Courtesy of* Lawrence Fung, DDS, Culver City, CA.)

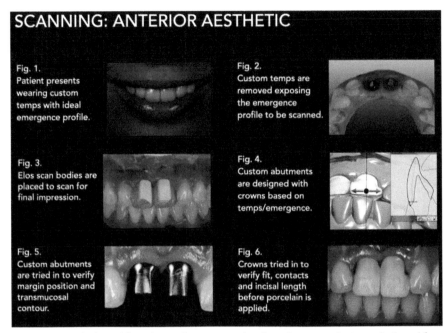

Fig. 14. Surgical plan with an immediate custom healing abutment that was designed from the preplanned implant coordinates.

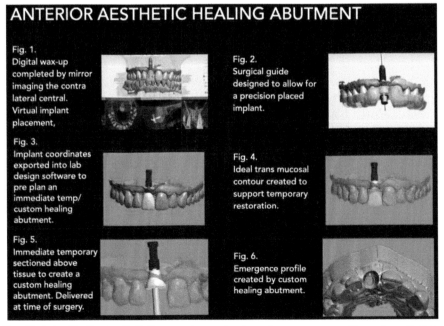

Fig. 15. It is effective to digitally record a predeveloped emergence profile and use that information to design the most ideal custom abutment and restoration.

and form the tissue profile that will aid in the development of papilla and is easily modified by simply adding composite if the transmucosal design requires modification.

In **Fig. 15**, it can be seen how effective it is to digitally record a predeveloped emergence profile and use that information to design the most ideal custom abutment and restoration.

In summary, digital dentistry could be a great addition to any practice. It does, however, have its drawbacks that need to be thoroughly understood. The digital process and workflows could be superior to conventional techniques in some respects, but the practitioner must be motivated to create systems in place to maximize the benefit of digital technology in the practice.

Incorporating a digital workflow into a dental environment is a daunting task. Whether in a clinical or laboratory environment, workflow options are endless, and the variety of technology is vast. The benefits of using technology are clear: increased levels of communication, predictability, and improved patient care.

DISCLOSURE

L. Fung, DDS is a paid consultant for SprintRay 3D printing technologies. P. Brisebois has nothing to disclose.

REFERENCES

1. Zaruba M, Mehl A. Chairside systems: a current review. Int J Comput Dent 2017; 20(2):119–213. Available at: https://www.quintessence-partner.com/chairside-systems-current-review.
2. Mangano F, Gandolfi A, Luongo G, et al. Intraoral scanners in dentistry: a review of the current literature. BMC Oral Health 2017;17(1):149.
3. All3DP. SLA vs DLP: the differences – simply explained. Available at: https://all3dp. com/2/dlp-vs-sla-3d-printing-technologies-shootout/. Accessed October 12, 2019.

FURTHER READINGS

Ender A, Mehl A. Influence of scanning strategies on the accuracy of digital intraoral scanning systems. Int J Comput Dent 2013;16:11–21.

Gurrea DDS. Evaluation of dental shade guide variability using cross-polarized photography. Int J Periodontics Restorative Dent 2016;36:e76–81.

Hegenbarth EA. Esthetics and Shade Communication: A Practical Approach. Eur J Esthet Dent 2006;1(4):p340–60.

Reshad M, Cascione D, Magne P. Diagnostic mock-ups as an objective tool for predictable outcomes with porcelain laminate veneers in esthetically demanding patients: a clinical report. J Prosthet Dent 2008;99:333–9.

Robertson AJ, Toumba KJ. Cross-polarized photography in the study of enamel defects in dental paediatrics. J Audiov Media Med 1999;22(2):63–70.

Sancho-Puchades M, Fehmer V, Hämmerle C, et al. Advanced smile diagnostics using CAD/CAM mock-ups. Int J Esthet Dent 2015;10:374–91.

Seelbach P, Brueckel C, Wöstmann B. Accuracy of digital and conventional impression techniques and workflow. Clin Oral Investig 2013;17:1759–64.

SLA vs DLP: the differences- simply explained. By Ricardo Pires. 2019. Available at: https://all3dp.com/2/dlp-vs-sla-3d-printing-technologies-shootout/.

The Use of Botulinum Toxin and Dermal Fillers to Enhance Patients' Perceived Attractiveness

Implications for the Future of Aesthetic Dentistry

Phong Tran Cao, DDS[a,b,]*

KEYWORDS

- Aesthetic dentistry • Cosmetic dentistry • Aesthetic medicine • Botox
- Dermal fillers

KEY POINTS

- Physical beauty has long held an important place in society, because of biologic and psychological predispositions to treat those one deems attractive in more positive ways.
- Facial features change over time and often represent the first and most obvious evidence of physical aging.
- Veneers and crowns, along with invasive surgical procedures, have previously been the only tools available to alter a patient's facial appearance and combat signs of aging.
- Today, aesthetic dentists have other means at their disposal, including Botox and dermal fillers, to greatly improve the appearance of their patients. These injectable products serve a complementary role to standard equipment in the dentist's armamentarium.

The field of aesthetic dentistry evolves with each passing day. New practices, products, devices, and perspectives continue to emerge, and dentists are leading the charge to change lives through a tailored approach that combines these elements to suit the unique needs of each individual patient. Although some may consider "changing lives" hyperbolic coming from a dentist's mouth, there is ample evidence indicating that a person's appearance can heavily impact his or her life experiences, and that a healthy, beautiful smile alone may achieve this.[1] Bearing this in mind,

[a] University of California, Los Angeles, Los Angeles, CA, USA; [b] Cosmetic Dentist and Private Practice, 5 Star Dental, 700 East Silverado Ranch Boulevard, Suite 100, Las Vegas, NV 89183, USA
* Cosmetic Dentist and Private Practice, 5 Star Dental, 700 East Silverado Ranch Boulevard, Suite 100, Las Vegas, NV 89183.
E-mail address: info@5star-dental.com

Dent Clin N Am 64 (2020) 659–668
https://doi.org/10.1016/j.cden.2020.06.003
0011-8532/20/© 2020 Elsevier Inc. All rights reserved.

dental.theclinics.com

aesthetic dentists who dedicate themselves to improving patients' smiles now have a unique opportunity to expand beyond the lower third of the face when addressing facial appearances. This opportunity comes in the form of such products as botulinum toxin (BTN) and fillers (eg, hyaluronic acid). Once limited to cosmetic surgeons' practices, these products also can aid dentists in addressing the aesthetic goals of their clients.

When considering the future of aesthetic dentistry and how best to help patients navigate their journey to a more attractive physical appearance, it is vital to understand the underlying reasons for humans' preoccupation with appearance and what is considered generally attractive. It is also necessary to question whether dentists are optimally using all tools and approaches at their disposal to support patients, and whether new and emerging treatments beyond the typical veneers and facial surgeries might offer a viable path forward. Dentists have a duty to improve not just their patients' smiles, but also their quality of life. Understanding and assisting aesthetic dental patients in their pursuit of a more attractive appearance is central to this role.

WHY ARE HUMANS SO PREOCCUPIED WITH PERCEIVED ATTRACTIVENESS?

The global beauty market is a billion-dollar business that is only expected to grow. The reason for this continued growth has ancient and modern roots.

Artists, such as Leonardo DaVinci, studied faces to discern ideal proportions, and the Roman poet Ovid wrote the first known manual of beauty advice for women. These creatives were studying attractiveness from a unique perspective and even today researchers continue to explore the concept of perceived attractiveness.

If history did not offer enough evidence to persuade one that humans are preoccupied with attractiveness, it should be noted that evolutionary theories, such as those regarding the survival of the fittest, also emphasize physical appearance. In fact, there is evidence that people look for symmetry or absence of gross asymmetry as a measure of health and fitness in a mate.[2]

Furthermore, evolutionary psychology tells us that males are attracted to traits associated with estrogen, such as bigger eyes and fuller lips or a smaller chin and more diminutive nose. And research finds that males also favor high cheekbones in women to indicate childbearing maturity. It is not only males who evaluate perceived attractiveness with an evolutionarily modified lens. Females look for traits synonymous with the presence of testosterone, such as square chins, broad musculature, and heavy brows.[3,4]

Aside from the general selection of a mate based on innate measures of perceived attractiveness, humans also make important decisions based on appearance. These decisions, research indicates, may mean that humans are predisposed to equate someone's personality or trustworthiness with one's perception of their facial aesthetic.

More visually pleasing or attractive faces may lead to different outcomes for those who have them and there is evidence that humans may consider attractive people morally superior, give them better grades in school, and even offer them a lighter punishment for crimes committed.[5,6]

Those considered attractive often experience greater employment success and find themselves being higher paid. Moreover, those who find themselves to be beautiful also judge themselves more favorably.[5,6]

Conversely, those with facial asymmetry or other atypical facial features may find themselves enduring a different set of social experiences. Those with facial asymmetry or facial features outside of the norm may be deemed untrustworthy, lazy, or less intelligent. Research indicates that these are not simply an indication of one's "preferences" from moment to moment. Studies indicate that the brain is essentially hardwired to perceive attractiveness in this light.[7]

Furthermore, there is evidence that humans view attractive faces differently, even from birth, and that this reaction is biologic and rapid. In fact, research indicates that infants respond to more attractive faces.[1] When humans are viewing an attractive face the fusiform gyrus that handles facial recognition activates the nucleus accumbens, the brain's reward center. It also stimulates activity in the amygdala where humans handle emotional responses. The frontal cortex, which is related to higher-order reasoning, is also impacted as is the orbitofrontal cortex, which handles decision making. Finally, activity is also present in the caudate nucleus, which formulates and activates repetitive or stereotyped behavioral responses when viewing attractive faces.

This chain of events indicates that the human body has an innate propensity to react to a face it perceives to be attractive by sending multiple rewarding signals to our brain. The brain receives these signals and begins a chain-reaction-like process of stimulation. As a result of this stimulation and that process, the brain can begin formulating and reinforcing stereotypes.

Those stereotypes, because of that reward system that is activated, become hardwired and cause humans to equate perceived attractiveness with positive emotions. There is also reason to believe that although the process is multifaceted, it occurs quickly: The brain can recognize and determine attractiveness in less than 13 milliseconds.[8,9]

ATTRACTIVENESS AND BEAUTY IN THE AGE OF SOCIAL MEDIA

With the advent of the Internet and the rise of social media, basic concepts of attractiveness have become heavily influenced by what is popular nationally and globally. Influencers, movie and television stars, pop culture icons, and the likes have all impacted what the general population considers attractive. The pervasive reach of the Internet has led to a propagation of norms of attractiveness, and those norms are now more easily recognizable than ever. The results of this phenomenon are a homogenization of beauty standards, because those on the receiving end seek to alter their own appearance to emulate that of their idols.

Although beauty norms are impacted by popular culture, there is still evidence that the general population leans on an evolutionarily predisposed ideal for attractiveness that includes facial symmetry, plump lips, and full cheeks. Finally, the obsession with youthfulness, which dates back to antiquity and is alive and well today, dictates a large part of today's beauty standards. Thus, traits that betray the process of aging, such as wrinkles, marionette lines, or jowls, are considered undesirable. Dentists, who spend their professional lives working in and around the mouth and the face, are more than familiar with signs of extreme aging.

SIGNS OF AGING: THE SKELETON AND FAT PAD ATROPHY

The human skeleton changes throughout its life via osteoblastic and osteoclastic activities. Patients in their twenties have skulls that are at their densest and as aging progresses, the skull morphs, leading to adjustments in one's facial appearance. These ongoing skeletal changes impact the overlying soft tissue, the skeletal muscle attachments, and the ligaments (**Fig. 1**).

In addition, the body's process of storing and distributing fat changes with aging. The compartmentalized fat pads that once gave babies their plump cheeks and held up the skin tautly begin to lose volume, and gaps develop between different

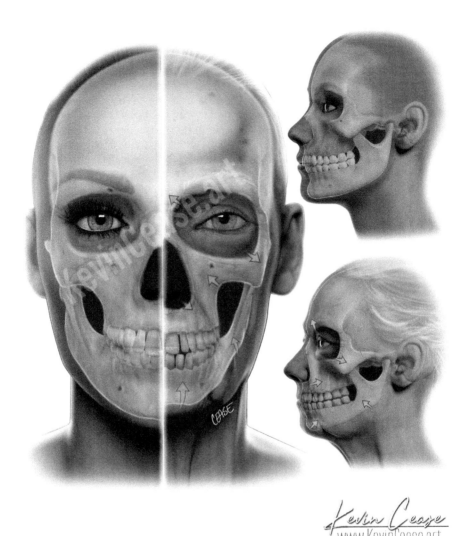

Fig. 1. Facial bone changes over time. (© 2020 Kevin Cease. All rights reserved.)

compartments. These changes are magnified by gravitational pull and a concurring loss of collagen in the skin, leading to weaker, less elastic skin. Taken together, these physical changes lead to an altered facial appearance, commonly described as sunken or uneven, that is indicative of aging.[10]

Additional changes occur with fat pads around the temporal fossa (**Fig. 2**). As they atrophy, temporal hollowing develops, compromising the integrity and support they have provided to the skin. The result is a sagging of the skin that contributes to the drooping of the lateral eyebrow to or below the level of the superior orbital rim; this sinking can occur in one or both orbital rims with age.[11] With more advanced aging, the appearance of wrinkles, hollowed cheeks, malar bags, and jowls provide further evidence of the deterioration of fat pads over time.

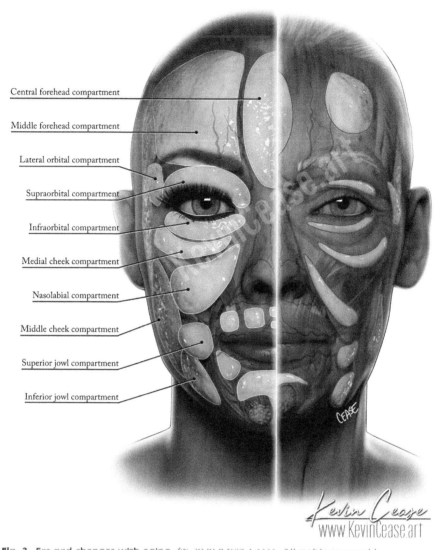

Fig. 2. Fat pad changes with aging. (© 2020 Kevin Cease. All rights reserved.)

CHANGES IN THE PERIORBITAL CAVITY AND MANDIBLE AS AN INDICATOR OF AGING

When discussing signs of aging, one cannot overlook the periorbital cavity. The periorbital cavity expands with time but not always in the same way. The changes to the inferolateral orbital rim occur by middle age, whereas those to the superomedial rim lag in time. Both, however, experience greater bone resorption than the remaining aspects of the orbital rim. Moreover, the infraorbital fat pad loses its integrity, forming an indentation that becomes more pronounced over time.

The jaw bone, anterior nasal spine, and pyriform aperture recede with age for patients who have teeth and those who no longer do.[12] This posterior movement is accompanied by a displacement of the soft tissue that lays over each.

These collective movements, coupled with the atrophy that occurs in the nasolabial fat pad, create a fold in the nasolabial region of the face. Furthermore, when the anterior nasal spine recedes backward, the columella also recedes. The result is that the nose tips downward and can appear longer than it had before.

The mandible itself undergoes some changes with age that can impact a patient's appearance. The ramus experiences a shortening effect and the chin bone is resorbed. The mandible's measurements are reduced with aging, in height and in length. The resorption of the mandible's prejowl area creates a concave shape that does not offer enough support for the overlying soft tissues in that area. The result is often a less defined jawline, evidence of jowls, and further indication of aging.[13] These changes beneath the skin can impact the superficial appearance of the face at the skin level (**Fig. 3**).

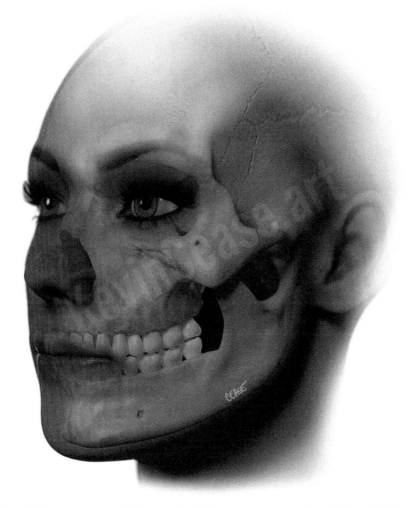

Fig. 3. The appearance of skin over skull. Changes happening beneath the skin change the superficial appearance of the skin. (© 2020 Kevin Cease. All rights reserved.)

AESTHETIC DENTISTRY APPROACHES TO ADDRESSING AGING AND IMPROVING PERCEIVED ATTRACTIVENESS

Dentists are able to enhance a patient's personal appearance, and aesthetic dentistry has been tasked with this mission since its inception. In general, dentists find themselves working within the lower third of the face, working to provide a full, bright, and beautiful smile to patients who seek dental care. Those who perform aesthetic dentistry procedures may work to reduce excessive buccal corridors by combining orthodontic treatment and veneers. The goal, in this case, is to provide support for a patient's hollow cheeks and the results would ideally be a more youthful and plump cheek appearance and symmetry.

Dentists may also work to enhance facial appearance by adjusting the height of the lower third of the face. This may mean increasing the vertical dimension of occlusion or using orthognathic surgery to decrease that same section. The result, in either case, would be to address protrusion or recession and achieve the desired facial aesthetic for the patient.

OTHER POTENTIAL MEASURES TO IMPACT A PATIENT'S PERCEIVED ATTRACTIVENESS

Aside from the aforementioned dental procedures, dentists have access to other tools that can support patients in achieving their aesthetic dentistry goals. In recent years, facial injections, such as the neurotoxin BTN, and facial fillers, such as hyaluronic acid, previously reserved for the cosmetic surgeon and aesthetician's practice have become available to other specialties. Indeed, a growing number of states have extended the approved use of these dermal fillers and injections to include provisions that allow dentists to offer these services to their patients in the dental office. This affords dentists the chance to further help patients achieve their aesthetically related treatment goals.

BOTULINUM TOXIN

BTN is produced by the obligate anaerobic bacterium *Clostridium botulinum*. At a basic chemical level, BTN consists of a light chain and a heavy chain connected by a disulfide bond. The heavy chain has a high affinity for nerve terminals that uptake acetylcholine, and is responsible for BTN entering the neuron through endocytosis. Once inside, the light chain becomes detached from the heavy chain, infiltrates outside the vesicle membrane, and targets the snare protein cleaving part of the SNAP25 protein. This prevents the acetylcholine vesicles from binding to the presynaptic receptor, blocking the release of a signal that would cause muscle contraction. This leads to localized paralysis. Once the SNAP25 protein is destroyed, it is no longer able to release the neurotransmitter responsible for contraction. When practitioners who inject BTN target specific muscles, the result is a smoothing and relaxing of the skin, and reduction if not effacement of wrinkles.

There is also evidence that BTN may be beneficial for the treatment of myofascial pain, bruxism, and controlling the occlusal force.[14] Furthermore, because myofascial pain is often associated with the constant contraction of particular muscle groups, practitioners can target these trigger points to impact the pain pathway and interfere with the way pain travels to other parts of the patient's body.[14]

HYALURONIC ACID

Hyaluronic acid is a clear gel-like polysaccharide substance found in the human body. It is a nonsulfated glycosaminoglycan distributed throughout the connective, epithelial, and neural tissues (see **Fig. 1**). Hyaluronic acid is highly hydrophilic in nature and helps lubricate joints and allows the skin to appear smooth.

Most hyaluronic acid fillers that are used in aesthetic medicine are derived from bacterial cultures. Hyaluronic acid molecules are typically cross-linked to slow down the degenerative process. The advantage of hyaluronic acid fillers is that their effects are reversible with the use of hyaluronidase. Because vessel occlusion is not an uncommon scenario, it is common best practice to keep the antidote on hand when offering hyaluronic acid fillers. The manner in which hyaluronic acid fillers are applied significantly impacts the results. Placing these fillers under the skin can result in hydrated, plump skin appearance, which is often considered a sign of youthfulness. When hyaluronic acid fillers are placed with care and strategy under certain muscle groups or on bone, they can support and alter the location of the skin.[15,16] Hyaluronic acid and dermal fillers can also be used to address hollowing of the cheeks.

USE OF HYALURONIC ACID AND BOTULINUM TOXIN IN AESTHETIC DENTISTRY
Occlusal Force

Aesthetic dentists understand that each patient's characteristics demand an individualized approach. Controlling for the occlusal force, for example, remains a great challenge. A dentist may provide well-designed veneers or crowns but cannot account for occlusal force acting on those prostheses over time. These long-lasting procedures are impacted by a patient's propensity to wear down teeth or to develop masseter hypertrophy. In addition, patients' compliance is also a challenge in this area, and BTN may be a remedy for this issue. Injecting the masseter muscle with BTN may lead to a slimming of the face or jawline through atrophy of the masseter muscle, which may also impact occlusal force.[14,15]

Black Triangle

Black triangle or loss of interdental papillae volume is another challenge that aesthetic dentists face when working with patients. Although a common approach to the black triangle is to adjust the shape of the patient's teeth, hyaluronic acid fillers may also be a helpful measure. The filler is highly effective in treating black triangles when injected directly into the papillae. This causes the area to plump up and can minimize the void or black triangle.[17]

Gummy Smile

Another common cosmetic challenge dentist's face is the gummy smile. A gummy smile is usually the result of an amalgamation of several factors, including a thin upper lip, gingival hyperplasia, the skeletal position of the maxilla, delayed passive eruption, and labial hypermobility. If a patient has a minor gummy smile, fillers are used to increase the volume of their lips. This volume decreases the amount of gingival display and can enhance the overall appearance of the smile.

A gummy smile can also be addressed by targeting the levator labii superioris alaeque nasi and the levator labii superioris located lateral to the alae of the nose. In so doing, practitioners weaken the elevation of those muscles and correct the hypermobility of the lip, thereby correcting the gummy smile.

SUMMARY AND IMPLICATIONS FOR FUTURE PRACTICE

Given the deeply ingrained evolutionary, social, psychological, and biologic forces driving the pursuit of a more appealing physical appearance, patients will continue to seek out the assistance of aesthetic dentists and clinicians to help them attain some personal measure of improved beauty. This desire to appear more attractive is indeed deeply human. It dates back to the beginning of mankind; it is enduring and will continue to grow throughout our existence. It is central to the craft and profession of aesthetic dentists.

In the past, dentists who wished to change their patients' appearance for the better were limited to addressing their teeth and smiles, working primarily with crowns, veneers, and mandibular adjustments or surgeries to achieve beneficial results. However, as more tools and options become available in this task, the dental profession will find itself faced with several decisions. It will need to decide whether as a community, it has the obligation to learn to use these tools, and how best to apply them in the service of patients. It will also need to decide if dentists should seize this opportunity to move toward addressing the upper two-thirds of the patient's face. Finally, the profession will need to decide if dentists should step forward to become a trusted source to guide the use of new and emerging science and tools.

Two such tools relevant to aesthetic dentistry are hyaluronic acid and BTN. In both cases, the field should take note. BTN is used to address facial tensing related to the constriction of muscles in the face and can reduce the appearance of fine lines and wrinkles. Hyaluronic acid may be used to plump and smooth the appearance of skin leading to a more youthful appearance. These tools are already in use in dental offices across the country, and their application will only continue to grow as word of their effectiveness reaches even more patients. Whether it is through relief of pain, reduction of sagging and plumping in the skin, and easing of wrinkles, these two tools have been shown to create youthful, attractive, and positive results for patients who receive them.

In a society preoccupied with physical appearance, it is conceivable, and becoming more commonplace, that dentists will find themselves asked by patients not only for a new and brighter smile, but also for a remedy to their sagging wrinkles and aging facial features. Although cosmetic surgeons and other professionals may be able to offer these services to their patients, dentists are uniquely positioned to be of service in this area in a comprehensive way. Patients may purposefully seek out their dental professionals specifically because dentists know the face intimately and study it rigorously, and because their unique area of expertise, the smile, rests at the core of an attractive face. A dentist's years of training and practice may give patients confidence in his or her ability to safely and effectively offer BTN and hyaluronic acid fillers.

It bears mentioning that dentists need not ignore or overlook the use of veneers, crowns, or even orthodontia. In fact, in some cases, it may be preferable to resort to one of these approaches instead of BTN or hyaluronic acid fillers. However, arming themselves with a wide array of options allows dentists to offer the most appropriate and impactful treatment to each patient based on his or her unique needs. These products may be combined with a full array of other relevant approaches. The goal remains the same: to provide the best possible care and achieve the best possible outcome for each patient.

As aesthetic dentistry continues to evolve, it is imperative that dentists consider how adoption and incorporation of these tools can change the lives of their patients and how it may help shape the future of the profession.

DISCLOSURE

The author has nothing to disclose.

REFERENCES

1. Slater A. Visual perception in the newborn infant: issues and debates. Intellectica 2002;34(1):57–76.
2. Møller AP, Swaddle JP. Asymmetry, developmental stability, and evolution. Oxford (United Kingdom): Oxford Univ. Press; 2002.
3. Fink B, Penton-Voak IS. Evolutionary psychology of facial attractiveness. Curr Dir Psychol Sci 2002;11:154–8.
4. Smith ML, Perrett D, Jones B, et al. Facial appearance is a cue to estrogen levels in women. Proc R Soc B Biol Sci 2005;273(1583):135–40.
5. Biddle J, Hamermesh D. Beauty, productivity and discrimination: lawyers looks and lucre. 1995. https://doi.org/10.3386/w5366.
6. Langlois JH, Kalakanis L, Rubenstein AJ, et al. Maxims or myths of beauty? A meta-analytic and theoretical review. Psychol Bull 2000;126(3):390–423.
7. Chatterjee A, Vartanian O. Neuroscience of aesthetics. Ann N Y Acad Sci 2016;1369(1):172–94.
8. Olson IR, Marshuetz C. Facial attractiveness is appraised in a glance. Emotion 2005;5(4):498–502.
9. Cloutier J, Heatherton TF, Whalen PJ, et al. Are attractive people rewarding? Sex differences in the neural substrates of facial attractiveness. J Cogn Neurosci 2008;20(6):941–51.
10. Mendelson B, Wong C-H. Changes in the facial skeleton with aging: implications and clinical applications in facial rejuvenation. Aesthetic Plast Surg 2012;36(4):753–60.
11. Coleman S, Grover R. The anatomy of the aging face: volume loss and changes in 3-dimensional topography. Aesthet Surg J 2006;26(1). https://doi.org/10.1016/j.asj.2005.09.012.
12. Pessa JE. An algorithm of facial aging: verification of Lambros's Theory by three-dimensional stereolithography, with reference to the pathogenesis of midfacial aging, scleral show, and the lateral suborbital trough deformity. Plast Reconstr Surg 2000;106(2):479–88.
13. Shaw RB, Katzel EB, Koltz PF, et al. Aging of the mandible and its aesthetic implications. Plast Reconstr Surg 2010;125(1):332–42.
14. Zhang L-D, Liu Q, Zou D-R, et al. Occlusal force characteristics of masseteric muscles after intramuscular injection of botulinum toxin A (BTX – A) for treatment of temporomandibular disorder. Br J Oral Maxillofac Surg 2016;54(7):736–40.
15. Sewane S, Jadhao V, Lokhande N, et al. Efficacy of botulinum toxin in treating myofascial pain and occlusal force characteristics of masticatory muscles in bruxism. Indian J Dent Res 2017;28(5):493.
16. Maio MD. Myomodulation with injectable fillers: an innovative approach to addressing facial muscle movement. Aesthetic Plast Surg 2018;42(3):798–814.
17. Lee W-P, Seo Y-S, Kim H-J, et al. The association between radiographic embrasure morphology and interdental papilla reconstruction using injectable hyaluronic acid gel. J Periodontal Implant Sci 2016;46(4):277.

A Beginning Guide for Dental Photography

A Simplified Introduction for Esthetic Dentistry

David J. Wagner, DDS[a,b],*

KEYWORDS

- Dental photography • Beginner's guide • Esthetic dentistry

KEY POINTS

- Dental photography is a simple and available tool that can transform a dental practice.
- Dental photography is a skill that is needed in order to perform high-level, predictable esthetic dentistry.
- Dental photography plays a critical role in the continuous journey of self-improvement for esthetic dentists.

BEGINNING THE JOURNEY

My first introduction to dental photography was during my Advanced Education in General Dentistry residency at University of California, Los Angeles (UCLA) School of Dentistry. We were required to buy a simple digital single-lens reflex (DSLR) camera, macro lens, and ring flash. Looking back, I lacked a full understanding of photography concepts and its value for a dentist. I had a scarcity mindset: the goal was to spend the least amount of money while satisfying the program requirements, rather than to truly understand the process of dental photography and its value. I did not have a workflow. When my photos were of poor quality I was not sure why. When my photos were of good quality, I simply got lucky. I was learning a tremendous amount about complex restorative dentistry, implants, and esthetics, but I was not using my camera with intention as I do today. I did not fully understand the camera as a necessary instrument for the type of dentist I wanted to be: practicing esthetic, restorative, and comprehensive dentistry at the highest level possible.

Two things occurred in my career that shaped my path. First, I started a continuing education (CE) journey with purpose, seeking high-level courses that taught comprehensive, patient-centered, relationship-based approaches to dental care. These courses all used photography as the foundation upon which to build a relationship,

[a] Private Practice, West Hollywood, CA, USA; [b] UCLA Center for Esthetic Dentistry
* 8733 Beverly Boulevard #202, West Hollywood, CA 90048.
E-mail address: davidjohnwagner@gmail.com

Dent Clin N Am 64 (2020) 669–696
https://doi.org/10.1016/j.cden.2020.07.002
0011-8532/20/© 2020 Elsevier Inc. All rights reserved.

trust, and understanding with a patient as well as perform accurate diagnosis and form a treatment plan. Second, I started taking dental photography courses. Third, once some formal photography education was underway, I began teaching photography at the UCLA Center for Esthetic Dentistry. These experiences, and many hours to taking photos in a private setting, have shaped my ability to understand photography as it relates to dentistry. More importantly, it has allowed an evolution to continue to distill the complex into more and more simple workflows.

VALUE AND PURPOSE OF DENTAL PHOTOGRAPHY

- Documentation
- Patient education and case acceptance
- Collaborating and communication with colleagues
- Marketing and branding
- Dental education
- Evaluating outcomes

Documentation

Beyond esthetic dentistry, creating thorough records is imperative to operating a compliant and responsible practice. All new patients should have photographs taken of their starting condition as they enter the practice for clinical reference as well as medical-legal protection for the dentist. Initial photographs serve as a time stamp of the patient's existing state when they first become a patient. It is important that these photographs are of high quality and include multiple views of the patient's face, smile, and dentition. Furthermore, within dental esthetics, a workflow should be developed in order to provide consistent, high-level documentation throughout all stages of treatment, including follow-up.

Patient Education and Case Acceptance

Photography is an integral part of communicating with patients. It allows the dentist to show the patient the starting point, existing conditions, findings, simulated treatment options, and examples of finished procedures for understanding and motivation. When discussing esthetic treatment, it provides a conduit to clearly understand patient goals, and aspects of their smiles they do not like and would like to enhance. One approach developed by dentist Bob Barkley in the 1960s and still taught in highly regarded CE courses is the process of codiscovery.

This process involves dentist, patient, and photography, and results in the patients gaining a thorough understanding of the conditions of their dentition and oral health. Bob Barkley spoke to this issue brilliantly when he said, "No greater risk of failure can be run than that of attempting to use traditional patient management procedures in a health oriented restorative practice. Examining and treating a patient's mouth without prior attitudinal development is an error of omission for which the dentist pays handsomely with time, energy, stress, and money."[1] Photography is key for this process and results in the success of the attitudinal development of patients, where patients can see their dentition, begin to fully understand and take ownership of their conditions and problems, and strongly value high-level treatment.[1]

In dental esthetics, through the process of diagnosis, treatment planning, and digital smile design, photography is used to develop a clear path for a patient's treatment. A smile design and proposed outcome can be presented to a patient. A digital simulation of the outcome has a profound impact emotionally on patients because they are able to experience how esthetic dental treatment can influence their overall appearance.

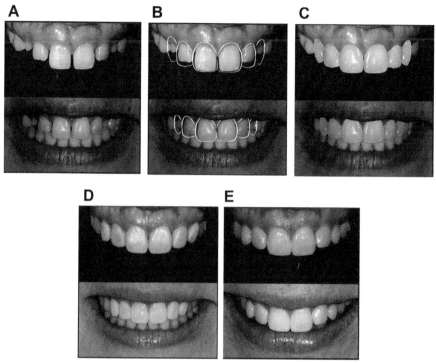

Fig. 1. (*A*) Initial Patient Presentation. (*B*) DSD Outline Form. (*C*) DSD Virtual Smile Simulation. (*D*) Prototype Try In based on Wax Up. (*E*) Final Restorations. (*Courtesy of* Yair Y. Whiteman, DMD, Los Angeles, CA.)

Fig. 1 shows the steps of a completed case motivated by photography and a digital smile design process. The more clinicians are able to communicate in this visual fashion, the more patients tend to understand their options and how esthetic dental treatment can help accomplish goals of improving their appearance.

Collaborating and Communication with Colleagues

Esthetic dental treatment is often interdisciplinary, involving close collaboration with other specialists. Esthetic dental treatment always requires detailed laboratory communication. Photography, presentation development, and digital smile design allows for optimal communication for interdisciplinary treatment planning to occur. If a dentist does not practice in close proximity to the dental lab that will be fabricating the restorations where a custom shade appointment can be accomplished, then photography will be required for shade matching purposes (**Fig. 2**). Photography is also used for evaluating restorations at the try-in appointment and then communicating to the laboratory if modifications are needed. Esthetic dental treatment cannot be done accurately or predictably without photography.

Branding and Marketing

Photography is needed when branding an esthetic dental practice as well as marketing the practice to both grow and maintain its relevance. Photography is used both internally and externally for these purposes. Before-and-after photos of patients can be shown to patients during a consultation. Specifically, completed treatments from

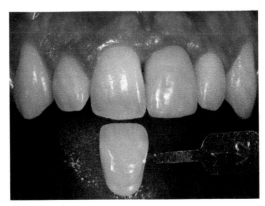

Fig. 2. Shade matching for esthetic treatment.

cases similar to a patient's condition can be used as a relatable example of someone else that underwent treatment and experienced an excellent outcome. Examples of completed cases should be included in your overall online presence to help patients find you for the type of treatment you are offering and they are seeking. Photography can help differentiate a dental practice from others depending on the quality that is performed and the style that is displayed.

Dental Education

Photography allows content development for lectures, study clubs, forums, and other aspects of education and collaboration among colleagues. When attending high-level dental meetings, incredible dental photography can be witnessed in presentations. Even if not currently teaching, documenting cases in a complete manner helps to build a library of content that may be used in the future should a teaching or lecturer position ever be pursued.

Evaluating Outcomes

Photography allows dentists to see the outcomes of their work as well as to evaluate successes and shortcomings.

> This is one of the most important factors for growth and development for practitioners of esthetic dentistry: every case, when documented well, scrutinized, and reviewed with colleagues and other experts, leads to exponential learning opportunities.

Routinely taking photographs at each step of treatment (diagnosis and treatment planning, prototype try-in, preparations, provisionals, final restoration try-in, cementation, and postoperative) collectively provides information that would otherwise not be available for fully understating outcomes, creating a path to mastering clinical skills.

PHOTOGRAPHY SETUP

Like other dental equipment and instrumentation, photography equipment comes in varying levels of quality and a wide range of price. So many options for photography equipment exists that it can be overwhelming for first-time users who are not sure where to start. Smartphones, point-and-shoot, and DSLR cameras are all options for the dentist and team. Although smartphones and point-and-shoot cameras are convenient, less expensive, and less technical, they do not have the overall functionality and nor do they produce the overall quality that DSLR cameras provide. Therefore, it is recommended that a DSLR camera be the primary camera for dental esthetics. There are multiple brand options for cameras and lighting that satisfy the level of quality desired; the aim of this guide is to simplify the shopping list with function, ease of use, and attainability in mind. There are five main categories encompassing proper photography setup:

DSLR camera body
Macro lens
Lighting setup
Accessories
Laptop computer

Digital Single-Lens Reflex Camera Body

The camera body is the main part of the camera minus the lens and lighting setup. Camera bodies come in 2 types: full frame and cropped sensor (Advanced Photo System type C [APS-C]). Full-frame cameras are what professional photographers use. Cropped-sensor cameras have a smaller sensor and are less expensive but are still of excellent quality. A full-frame camera will work for dental photography; however, a cropped-sensor camera is all that is needed for high-level dental photography. By choosing a cropped-sensor camera, a dentist can save thousands of dollars without sacrificing the quality that is needed. Because of their smaller sensors compared with full-frame cameras, APS-C cameras capture only part of the image produced by the lens. This feature is known as a crop factor.

To work around this small variation in sensor size (crop factor), the photographer simply needs to move slightly away from the subject to capture the same image at the same distance as a full-frame camera. This technique results in a magnification phenomenon that influences the focal length once the lens is connected to the body, which means that, depending on the space present in a dental practice, the proper lens type paired with a cropped-sensor camera allows the dentist to take photographs comfortably in a small operatory room setting, versus a larger studio space, which is not always available in a dental practice.

Macro Lens

The type of lens needed for dental photography is referred to as a macro lens. A lens is selected by brand, quality, focal length, and cost (**Table 1**). The lens is perhaps the most important aspect of the photography setup, where its physical quality is a greater determining factor of overall photo quality outcome than other parts of the dental photography setup. The number on the side of the lens signifies the focal length of the lens. The focal length determines how close the dentist needs to be to the patient in order to capture the desired photo. The appropriate focal length for dental photography is a range (85–105 mm), depending on the type of camera as well as how much space is present in the dental operatory or studio setting.

As discussed previously in this article, a cropped-sensor camera has a multiplying effect (crop factor) of 1.5×. Therefore, an 85-mm macro lens placed on a cropped-sensor camera translates to a focal length of 127.5 mm (85 mm × 1.5). A 100-mm macro lens placed on a cropped-sensor camera translates to a focal length of 150 mm (100 mm × 1.5). The 85-mm lens (lighter, smaller, and less expensive

Table 1
Macro lens recommendations

Lens	Pro	Con
Nikon AF-S Micro Nikkor 85 mm f/3.5	• Lighter in weight • Smaller in size • Less expensive • Decreased working distance required compared with Nikon 105 mm	• Slight lower quality compared with Nikon 105 mm
Nikon AF-S Micro Nikkor 105 mm f/2.8	• High quality • Excellent optics • Smooth, fast focus	• Heavier in weight • Expensive • Larger in size • Increased working distance required compared with Nikon 85 mm
Tamron SP 90 mm f/2.8	• Excellent optics • Middle price range • Can work closer to patient than Nikon 105 mm	• Cannot get as close to patient as Nikon 85 mm
Tokina atx-i 100 mm f/2.8	• Least expensive • Excellent optics • Light in weight	• Slow focus speed may be off-putting and slows efficiency

compared with the 100-mm macro lens) therefore allows the dentist to be closer to the patient when taking photos. This closer proximity of the dentist to the patient has significant advantages for shorter individuals as well as those with space restrictions who will be taking all photos in a standard dental operatory versus a studio space within the dental office.

Lighting Setup

An understanding of how to use and manipulate light is perhaps the most technical and important aspect of learning to deliver predictable dental photography at a high level. There are multiple lighting configurations for dental photography. With each lighting configuration option comes advantages and disadvantages. Within these configurations, 2 major categories exist: on-camera lighting and off-camera lighting.

Lights used for high-level dental photography are called either speedlights or strobes. Speedlights are less expensive, battery powered, portable, and can be used on or off camera, whereas strobes are more expensive, more delicate, only used off camera, and most need to be plugged into an electrical outlet. Both speedlights and strobes can easily be purchased online or at a photography store. When speedlights are used on camera, they are held by an adjustable bracket that is attached to the bottom of the camera body (**Fig. 3**). Multiple options for brackets to hold speedlights for on-camera lighting are available online. When speedlights or strobes are used off camera, they are positioned on a stand near the patient. These stands can easily be purchased online or at a local camera store.

A commander is the required piece of equipment that allows communication between the camera and the lights. The commander is also responsible for controlling the flash power, or the amount of light output each time the light flashes. In photography, the nomenclature used for flash power on both a commander and light source

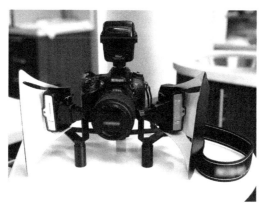

Fig. 3. Camera setup.

is as follows: 1:1 for full power, 1:2 for half power, 1:4 for one-quarter power, 1:8 for one-eighth power, and so on. Depending on the needs of the dental photographer, different levels of flash power may be used. Although some cameras have a built-in internal commander, it is recommended to use an external commander attached to the top of the camera for efficiency reasons, because the settings can be quickly viewed and changed on the commander display (see **Fig. 3**).

Light Modification

Light in flash photography can be modified from its original state to produce a superior image. Light is changed by forcing it to pass through a medium or directing the light elsewhere (filtering or scattering the light particles) before it reaches the subject. The process of filtering and scattering the light decreases the concentration of light particles and therefore results in what is referred to as modified light. An example of this is a reflector, diffusor, bouncer, or soft box that can be used in conjunction with speedlights and strobes (see **Fig. 3**). One elegant do-it-yourself approach to light modification that is commonly used is white paper stock placed in front of speedlights to function as a diffusor, which can function exactly like more expensive light modification equipment to create a more pleasing image (**Fig. 4**).

Unmodified light is typically described as harsh, creating undesired reflections that can block critical detail. Light that is modified by a diffusor or bouncer is described as soft, which produces more pleasing images. For example, in close-up photography, diffused light can help produce desired reflections that highlight nuances of teeth characterization, such as line angles and incisal translucency. In portrait photography, diffused light produces images with more flattering features, such as smoother skin, creating an overall more professional-looking and emotionally charged image. Note that, when using modifiers, additional flash power may be needed, or camera settings changed, to allow more light to the camera sensor, compared with settings without modifiers, in order to achieve an image with proper exposure. Light modifiers (reflectors, diffusors, bouncers, soft boxes) can easily be purchased online.

> Ring lights, a type of speedlight where the lights are concentrated at the edge of the lens, are a common type of light used in dental photography. However, these lights are better suited for intraoral or surgical pictures and are not flexible for achieving high-level photos for all-around esthetic dentistry.

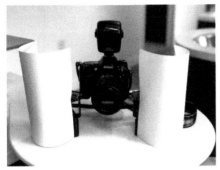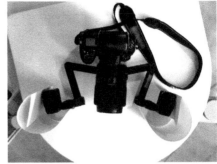

Fig. 4. Camera setup with white paper diffusors.

Light Arrangement

In photography, the position of the lights in relation to the subject influences the outcome of the image. Lights can be positioned closer to or farther from the lens as well as closer to or farther from the subject for both on-camera and off-camera lighting. Depending on the location of the lights, more or less highlight and shadow is created, leading to more or less depth. For clinical diagnostic photos, there should always be symmetrical lighting, where there is a lighting source on each side of the lens. For portrait photography, this rule does not always apply; depending on the type of image desired, a single light, either behind the photographer or off to one side of the subject, can result in slight shadowing on one side of the face. This shadowing creates a more interesting, dynamic image with additional depth and mood.

On-camera lighting position is changed by moving the speedlights attached to the adjustable bracket being used. Typically, lights are positioned next to the lens for intraoral photos and angled at 45° to the subject on each side for close-up smile photos and portraits.

Off-camera lighting with speedlights or strobes can be positioned in a similar fashion, either closer to the lens or at 45° angles to the subject. However, as mentioned before, often a single strobe with a soft box is appropriate for close-up smile or portrait when using strobe lighting. This single strobe light can be paired with a single reflector, or 2 reflectors (1 held by the patient). As mentioned before, reflectors are a form of light modification and help to bounce light and fill deficient areas, creating a more balanced and pleasing image. Note that certain strobe lights provide so much soft light that it can eliminate details of the teeth (commonly referred to as a washed-out appearance). It is often said that soft boxes can result in images that make the patient's restorations look like plastic denture teeth, which lack the vitality and sophistication of high-level, layered porcelain veneers. The type of lighting should be selected based on the intention of the clinician: diagnosis and treatment planning, documentation for patient education, building a before/after portfolio, or emotional images for branding and marketing.

Accessories

Various accessories are used in dental photography. **Table 2** includes a basic list. Additional accessories can be used depending on needs.

Laptop

In order to store, manage, edit, and present dental photography images, a computer is required. A laptop with photo editing software as well as presentation software is

Table 2 Accessories		
SD memory card	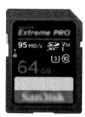	Multiple SD memory cards should be available. SD memory cards are reliable, but can easily become damaged, and therefore 64-GB memory capacity or less is an appropriate investment. Uploading photos to a hard drive and backup storage is recommend regularly, at least at the end of each clinical day
Lip retractors		Required to lift patient's lips away for intraoral photos. Can be metal or plastic. Metal is desired because plastic becomes scratched and faded easily when sterilized. Multiple sets of 2 should be sterilized together and kept packaged and ready for use
Occlusal mirrors (highlighted in yellow)		Paired with lip retractors, required for occlusal intraoral photos. Mirrors come in a variety of shapes and sizes, and additional accessories such as handles, for ease of use. Mirrors can be warmed to reduce fogging when in a patient's mouth. Stainless steel versions are available as well for a less fragile option. Proper handling and sterilizing reduces scratching and increases longevity
Buccal/lingual mirrors (highlighted in yellow)		Paired with lip retractors, required for buccal intraoral photos. Mirrors come in a variety of shapes and sizes, and additional accessories such as handles, for ease of use. Mirrors can be warmed to reduce fogging when in a patient's mouth. Stainless steel versions are available as well for a less fragile option. Proper handling and sterilizing reduces scratching and increases longevity
Black contraster		Paired with lip retractors, required to isolate areas of dentition (ie, maxillary anterior), moving lips out of the frame of the image and blocking out opposing dentition and other soft tissue. Comes in a variety of types and final photos will require editing in computer software

recommended, which can be easily used for putting together presentations for patients, specialists, and lectures. Note that dental photography images should not be manipulated so as to change reality; obtaining quality images with the camera itself is the goal, and simple cropping, rotating, and exposure changes can be accomplished with the computer software.

PHOTOGRAPHY CONCEPTS

Photography concepts must be understood in order to master dental photography. Understanding these concepts leads to understanding camera settings and therefore yields excellent photos: images that are in focus, have an appropriate depth of field, an accurate color tone, and proper exposure (**Table 3**).

Table 3
Photography concepts

Concept	Definition	Relationship	What It Means
Focal length	The distance from the glass of the lens to the sensor inside the camera body	The smaller the number, the wider the frame of the picture; 1.5× crop factor for DX (cropped-sensor cameras)	The smaller the number, the closer the dentist can get to a patient when taking photos
Aperture (f-stop)	The opening of the iris of the lens when taking a picture. Controlled and measured using f-stop. Regulates the amount of light that is allowed into the camera to the sensor	The lower the f-stop, the more light enters the camera The higher the f-stop, the less light enters the camera	A different f-stop is used for different types of dental photos. In general: f/11, portraits f/22, close-ups f/32, intraoral
Depth of field	What is in focus, influenced by the aperture (f-stop)	The higher the f-stop, the greater the depth of field. The lower the f-stop, the smaller the depth of field	A greater depth of field allows all teeth to be in focus from anterior to posterior
Shutter speed	Regulates the rate of opening of the iris, and thus the amount of light that enters the camera. Measured in fractions of a second	The slower the shutter speed, the more light enters the camera. The faster the shutter speed, the less light enters the camera	In dental photography, shutter speed is set at 1/125, and not changed; no need for adjustments
ISO	Measure of the sensitivity of the sensor to light. A digital sensor can be adjusted to be more or less sensitive by changing the ISO setting in the camera	The higher the ISO, the more sensitive the sensor is to light, and the brighter the picture. The lower the ISO, the less sensitive the sensor is to light, and the darker the picture	Because of a controlled environment with flashes in dental photography, ISO should be set at 100 or 200 and not changed. If ISO is too high, pictures get grainy with "noise"
White balance	The color balance on a digital camera. Can be adjusted depending on the lighting conditions or lights being used to give proper color balance	Measured in degrees Kelvin Low white balance results in more cool (blue) tones High white balance results in more warm (orange, red) tones	For most flash setups for dental photography, including the Nikon R1C1 speedlights, the white balance should be set at 5500 K. Other lighting setups may require different settings

Abbreviation: ISO, International Standards Organization.

Table 4	
f-Stop	
Type of Photograph	**F-stop**
Portrait	F10–F11
Close-up	F20–F25
Intraoral	F29–F32

Table 5		
Photography settings		
F-stop	F10–F32	Modify settings based on the type of photo being used
Shutter speed	1/125	Set and leave it. No need to change for dental photography
ISO	100–200	Set and leave it. May need to change between 100 and 200 if additional light is needed
White balance	5500 K	Set and leave it. Most lighting setups use 5500 K. Some require slight modification
Flash power	1:1, 1:2, 1:4	Set and leave it. May need to change if additional light is needed
Camera mode	Manual shooting mode	Set and leave it. No need to change for dental photography
Lens mode	Automatic or manual focus	Automatic focus is preferred for easy workflow. Manual focus may be used in extreme close-up situations where automatic focus is unable to function properly

PHOTOGRAPHY WORKFLOW AND SETTINGS

Once a camera is obtained, it is important to coordinate the camera settings to facilitate proper function for dental photography. Camera settings for dental photography are surprisingly simple: many are set once and not adjusted again. Other settings are modified easily and minimally based on workflow. An efficient way to develop a workflow is to change settings based on the type of images being captured. For the purposes of this article, three main categories of images are used in dental photography: portrait (full head); close-up (patient smiling, capture lips and some skin beyond the lips); intraoral (those taken with lip retractors, including facial, buccal, and occlusal views).

The most common setting to change is the f-stop, which regulates the aperture of the camera. For portrait images, the camera is farthest distance away from the patient, more light is required compared with close-up or intraoral images, and therefore a lower f-stop is appropriate. For portrait images, f-10 or f-11 should be used. For intraoral images, the camera is the closest to the patient, less light is required for a proper exposure, and therefore a higher f-stop is appropriate. For intraoral images, f-29 or f-32 should be used. Close-up images require a level of light in between portrait and intraoral images, and therefore an f-stop of 20 to 25 should be used (**Table 4**). The appropriate f-stop paired with other appropriate settings gives the proper exposure and depth of field for the image (**Table 5**).

Within the 3 main categories of photos, there are multiple images that should be obtained to acquire all views required for diagnosis and treatment planning and case work-up. An abbreviated set of images can be used based on needs. For example, fewer photos may be needed for a new patient with no treatment needs and images simply for initial documentation versus a patient with complex treatment needs, where all images should be taken for maximum visual data. Appendix 1 contains an image series outlining a recommended clinical workflow, illustrations for reference of position of patient and dentist, patient image examples of dental photographs, and associated camera settings. This guide can be copied and taken into the operatory for an easy reference. This workflow requires one photographer and one assistant. It is recommended that dentists master photography first and then they can train team members to take the dental photographs if competency can be achieved.

SUMMARY

Photography is a simple and available tool that, once mastered, can enable dentists to perform esthetic dentistry at the highest, most predictable level. However, photography is like other aspects of dentistry: it must be practiced over and over to reach a level where the dentist is confident and proficient to obtain excellent results every time. Photography allows patients to find and choose dental practices; without this, little esthetic dentistry will be done. Photography allows dentists to communicate to their patients what is possible and it allows the transfer of information among the entire team behind creating a new smile. Ultimately, photography allows the achievement of optimal clinical outcomes that will be life-changing for patients and plays a critical role in the continuous journey of self-improvement for esthetic dentists.

DISCLOSURE

The author has nothing to disclose.

REFERENCE

1. Codiscovery. Co-discovery and co-diagnosis: what's the difference?. Available at: https://codiscovery.com/paul-henny/co-discovery-co-diagnosis-whats-the-difference/. Accessed February 3, 2020.

APPENDIX 1:

Courtesy of David Wagner DDS, West Hollywood, CA

Complete Photo Series
[workflow for on camera flashes]

INTRAORAL
(USING RETRACTORS FOR ALL):

Patient in dental chair, reclined to 45 degrees.
Standing on patient's left side:

1) Right buccal, teeth together (buccal mirror)
2) Right buccal, teeth apart (buccal mirror)

Standing on patient's right side:

3) Left buccal, teeth together (buccal mirror)
4) Left buccal, teeth apart (buccal mirror)

Continue standing patient's right side, move dental chair flat:

5) Mandibular occlusal (occlusal mirror)

Move to standing behind patient, dental chair remains flat:

6) Maxillary occlusal (occlusal mirror)

7) Facial view, teeth together (no mirror)
8) Facial view, teeth apart (no mirror)
9) Facial view maxillary teeth only (Black Contraster)

CLOSE UP
(NO RETRACTORS)

Sitting in non dental chair at same level as the patient:

10) Frontal view: Natural smile
11) Frontal view: Full (maximum display) smile
12) Frontal view: Lips at rest

13) Right lateral view: Natural smile
14) Right lateral view: Full (maximum display) smile
15) Left lateral view: Natural smile
16) Left lateral view: Full (maximum display) smile

PORTRAIT [FULL FACE]
(WHITE OR BLACK BACKGROUND)

17) Frontal view: Natural smile
18) Frontal view: Full (maximum display) smile
19) Frontal view: Lips at rest
20) Frontal view: Retracted, teeth together
21) Frontal view: Retracted, teeth apart
22) Profile (side of face): Natural smile
23) Profile (side of face): Lips at rest
24) 12 O-Clock (head tipped forward)

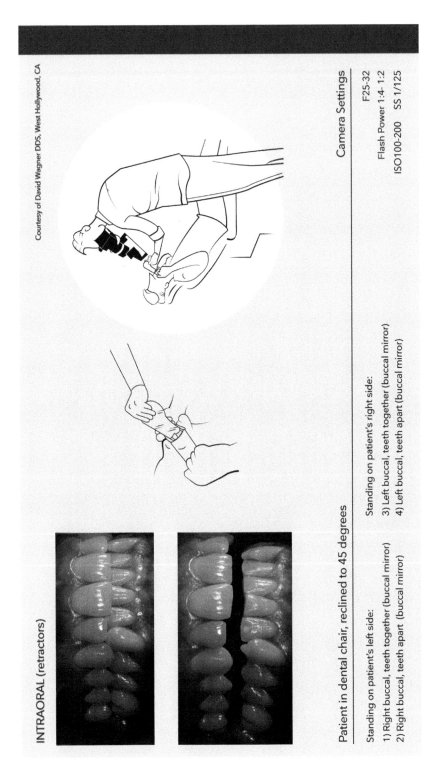

INTRAORAL (retractors)

Courtesy of David Wagner DDS, West Hollywood, CA

Camera Settings

F25-32
Flash Power 1:4- 1:2
ISO100-200   SS 1/125

Patient in dental chair, reclined to 45 degrees

Standing on patient's left side:
1) Right buccal, teeth together (buccal mirror)
2) Right buccal, teeth apart (buccal mirror)

Standing on patient's right side:
3) Left buccal, teeth together (buccal mirror)
4) Left buccal, teeth apart (buccal mirror)

INTRAORAL (retractors)

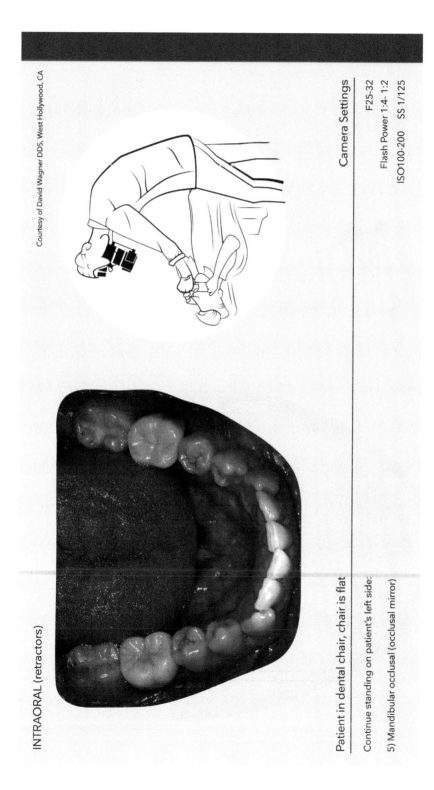

Courtesy of David Wagner DDS, West Hollywood, CA

Camera Settings

F25-32

Flash Power 1:4- 1:2

ISO100-200   SS 1/125

Patient in dental chair, chair is flat

Continue standing on patient's left side:

5) Mandibular occlusal (occlusal mirror)

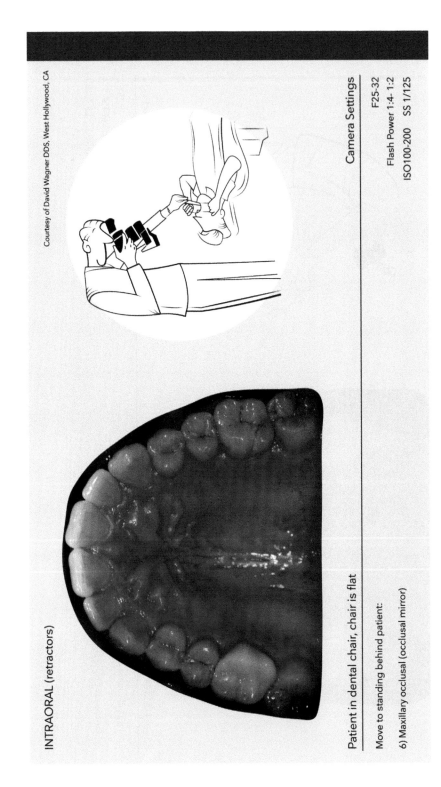

Courtesy of David Wagner DDS, West Hollywood, CA

INTRAORAL (retractors)

Camera Settings

F25-32
Flash Power 1:4- 1:2
ISO100-200   SS 1/125

Patient in dental chair, chair is flat

Move to standing behind patient:

6) Maxillary occlusal (occlusal mirror)

INTRAORAL (retractors)

Courtesy of David Wagner DDS, West Hollywood, CA

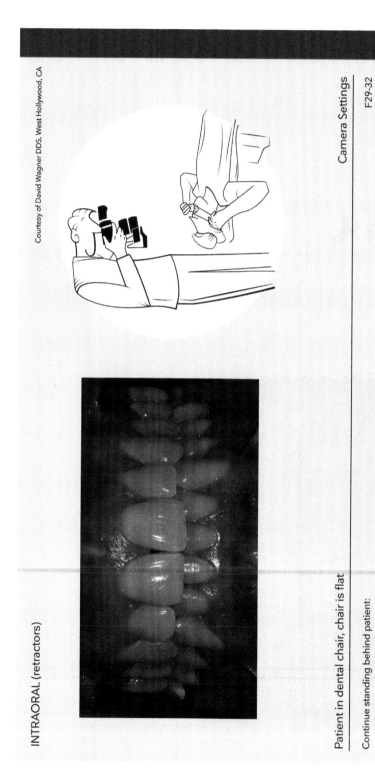

Camera Settings

F29-32

Flash Power 1:4- 1:2

ISO100-200   SS 1/125

Patient in dental chair, chair is flat

Continue standing behind patient:

7) Facial view, teeth together (no mirror)

INTRAORAL (retractors)

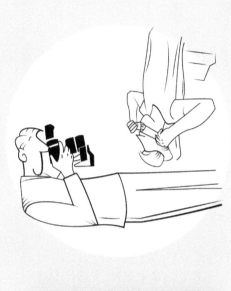

Courtesy of David Wagner DDS, West Hollywood, CA

Patient in dental chair, chair is flat

Continue standing behind patient:

8) Facial view, teeth apart (no mirror)

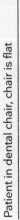

Camera Settings

F29-32
Flash Power 1:4- 1:2
ISO100-200   SS 1/125

INTRAORAL (retractors)

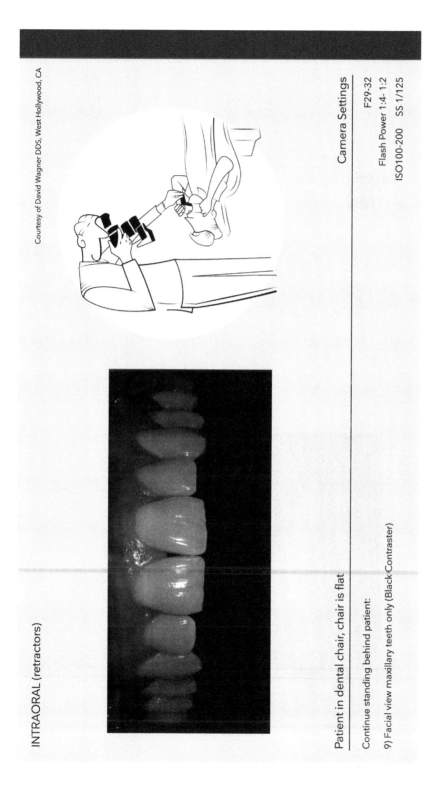

Courtesy of David Wagner DDS, West Hollywood, CA

Camera Settings

F29-32

Flash Power 1:4- 1:2

ISO100-200   SS 1/125

Patient in dental chair, chair is flat

Continue standing behind patient:

9) Facial view maxillary teeth only (Black Contraster)

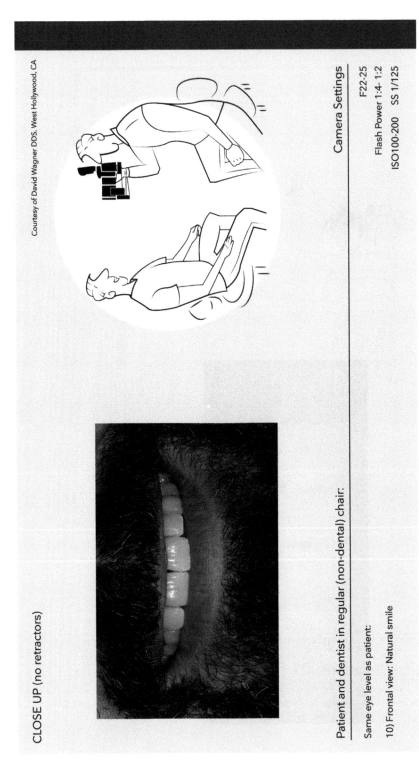

CLOSE UP (no retractors)

Courtesy of David Wagner DDS, West Hollywood, CA

Camera Settings

F22-25
Flash Power 1:4- 1:2
ISO100-200   SS 1/125

Patient and dentist in regular (non-dental) chair:

Same eye level as patient:

10) Frontal view: Natural smile

CLOSE UP (no retractors)

Courtesy of David Wagner DDS, West Hollywood, CA

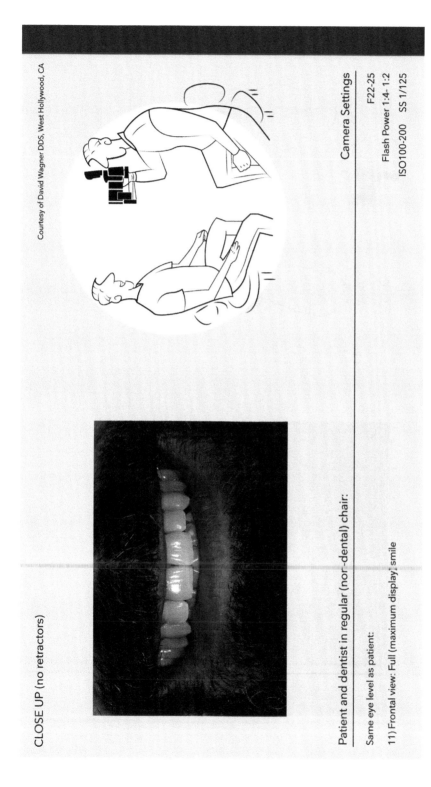

Patient and dentist in regular (nor-dental) chair:

Same eye level as patient:

11) Frontal view: Full (maximum display) smile

Camera Settings

F22-25

Flash Power 1:4- 1:2

ISO100-200   SS 1/125

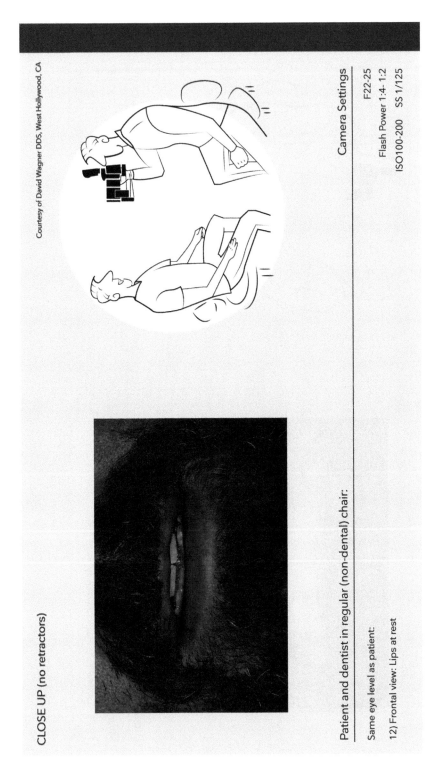

CLOSE UP (no retractors)

Courtesy of David Wagner DDS, West Hollywood, CA

Camera Settings

F22-25
Flash Power 1:4- 1:2
ISO100-200   SS 1/125

Patient and dentist in regular (non-dental) chair:

Same eye level as patient:

12) Frontal view: Lips at rest

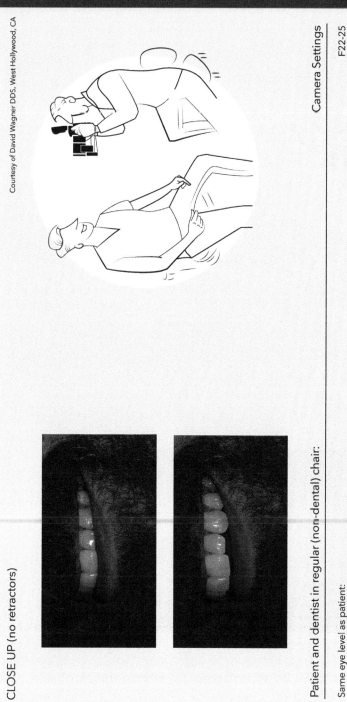

Courtesy of David Wagner DDS, West Hollywood, CA

Camera Settings

F22-25

Flash Power 1:4- 1:2

ISO100-200   SS 1/125

CLOSE UP (no retractors)

Patient and dentist in regular (non-dental) chair:

Same eye level as patient:

13) Right lateral view: Natural smile

14) Right lateral view: Full (maximum display) smile

15) Left lateral view: Natural smile

16) Left lateral view: Full (maximum display) smile

PORTRAIT (Full face)

Courtesy of David Wagner DDS, West Hollywood, CA

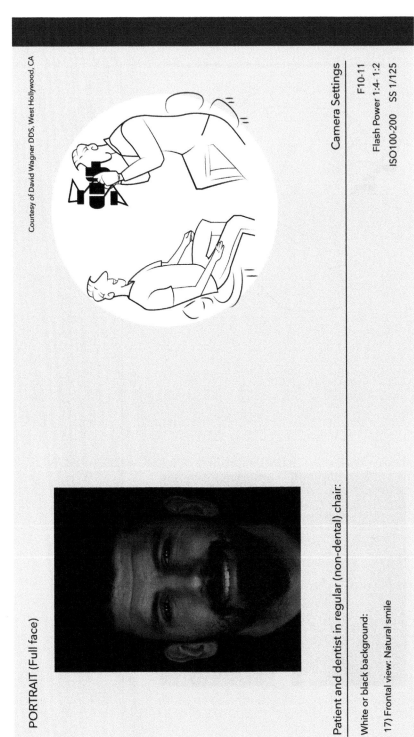

Camera Settings

F10-11
Flash Power 1:4- 1:2
ISO100-200   SS 1/125

Patient and dentist in regular (non-dental) chair:

White or black background:

17) Frontal view: Natural smile

PORTRAIT (Full face)

Courtesy of David Wagner DDS, West Hollywood, CA

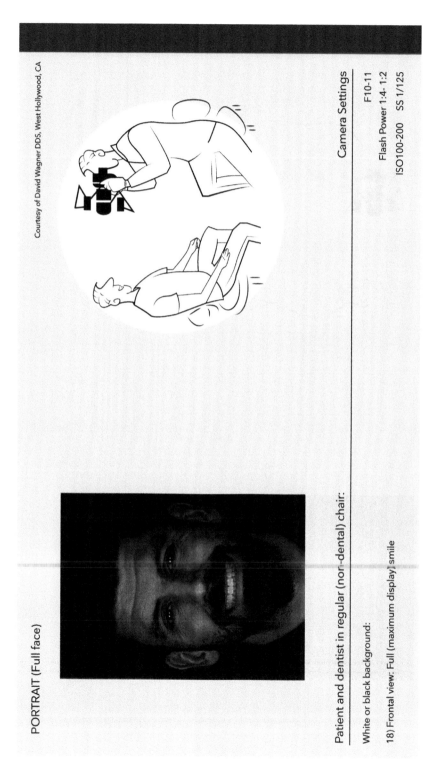

Patient and dentist in regular (non-dental) chair:

White or black background:

18) Frontal view: Full (maximum display) smile

Camera Settings

F10-11

Flash Power 1:4- 1:2

ISO100-200   SS 1/125

PORTRAIT (Full face)

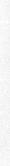

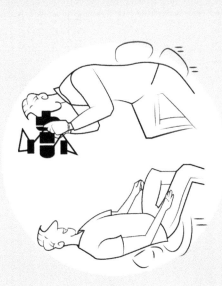

Patient and dentist in regular (non-dental) chair:

White or black background:

19) Frontal view: Lips at rest

Camera Settings

F10-11

Flash Power 1:4- 1:2

ISO100-200   SS 1/125

PORTRAIT (Full face)

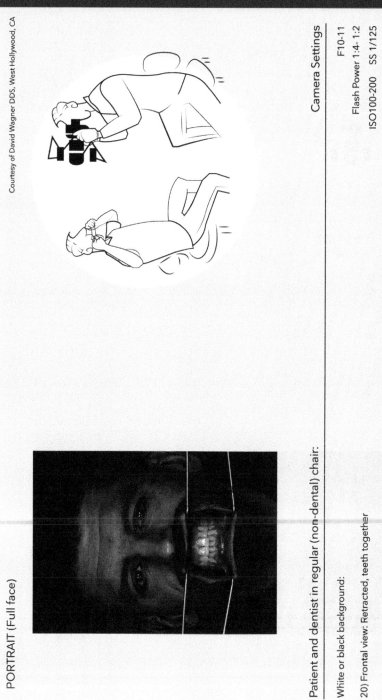

Courtesy of David Wagner DDS, West Hollywood, CA

Camera Settings

F10-11

Flash Power 1:4- 1:2

ISO100-200   SS 1/125

Patient and dentist in regular (non-dental) chair:

White or black background:

20) Frontal view: Retracted, teeth together

PORTRAIT (Full face)

Courtesy of David Wagner DDS, West Hollywood, CA

Patient and dentist in regular (non-dental) chair:

White or black background:

21) Frontal view: Retracted, teeth apart

Camera Settings

F10-11
Flash Power 1:4- 1:2
ISO100-200   SS 1/125

Courtesy of David Wagner DDS, West Hollywood, CA

Dentist-Ceramist Communication
Protocols for an Effective Esthetic Team

Sivan Finkel, DMD[a,b],*, Peter Pizzi, CDT, MDT[a,c]

KEYWORDS

- Communication • Photography • Smile design • Esthetic dentistry

KEY POINTS

- Close dentist/ceramist communication is critical for successful esthetic dentistry, and it is the dentist's responsibility to accurately convey the patient's desires to the ceramist.
- Digital photography is an indispensable tool for the esthetic dental team.
- Each patient should be analyzed from the facial (full face), dental-facial (lips and teeth), and dental (teeth only) perspectives.
- The most important element and starting point of any smile design is the three-dimensional position of the maxillary central incisor's incisal edge within the face.
- Whenever possible, an intraoral esthetic evaluation is performed at the outset. This evaluation serves to motivate the patient, identifies any potential limitations, and allows the team to assess the plan before performing any irreversible treatment.

Teamwork: the combined action of a group of people, especially when effective and efficient.

INTRODUCTION

No matter how skilled and well trained esthetic dentists or technicians may be, they cannot deliver results without a proper partnership. Close ceramist-clinician communication is a critical component of successful esthetic dentistry. In order to design an esthetic vision, convey this vision to the patient, and then execute the vision successfully, there must be effective communication between the ceramist, the clinician, and (most importantly) the patient.

[a] Advanced Program for International Dentists in Esthetic Dentistry, New York University College of Dentistry, New York, NY, USA; [b] The Dental Parlour, New York, NY, USA; [c] Pizzi Dental Studio, 4038 Victory Boulevard, Staten Island, NY 10314, USA
* Corresponding author. 434 East 57th Street, New York, NY 10022.
E-mail address: sivan@DentalParlourNYC.com
Instagram: @drsivanfinkel (S.F.)

Dent Clin N Am 64 (2020) 697–708
https://doi.org/10.1016/j.cden.2020.06.005
0011-8532/20/© 2020 Elsevier Inc. All rights reserved.

To execute high-level esthetics, both members of the dentist/technician team must have a deep understanding of tooth position, preparation design, form, color, and of the indications/limitations of the many materials available.

Although it is easy to connect with people via social media these days, if hoping to partner with a like-minded, serious counterpart, a beginning dentist or ceramist would be wise to attend symposiums and courses geared toward both groups. Aside from the quality of the lectures and educational value of these events, the networking element is equally important. Those who spend the time and money to travel to these sort of conferences and courses are serious about their profession. It is also inspiring and educational for anyone just starting out to rub shoulders with those who have already achieved greatness in the profession. As the saying goes, if you are the smartest person in the room, you are in the wrong room.

The authors of this article, both New Yorkers and both on New York University faculty, only met for the first time in California, during a conference's networking session 6 years ago. This article highlights some of the philosophies they share, as well as an overview of the key communication protocols that have proved effective for this team.

Philosophy

As restorative options evolve, our understanding of each material's optical and functional properties must evolve. Each patient presents unique challenges and the solution is never 1 size fits all. It is crucial for ceramists to be comfortable with a wide range of materials, and that clinicians understand the differences in preparation design and cementation that each material necessitates.

In terms of practicing conservative dentistry, the authors aim to be minimally invasive whenever possible, but with the understanding that some patients call for a less conservative approach. For example, a 0.3-mm porcelain veneer in a patient where the tooth substrate is extremely dark might not make as much sense as a full-coverage crown. The authors share the view that, in the words of Dr Marcelo Calamita, clinicians should be less concerned with minimal preparation and more concerned with appropriate preparation.[1]

Another viewpoint the authors share is that the ceramist must be involved from the beginning of each case, during the initial planning phase. Material considerations often have implications on not only the tooth preparations but also the surgical aspects of a case. A common example of this is situations where there is a soft tissue deficiency. The decision must be made at the outset whether the pink deficiency will be solved surgically (grafting) or prosthetically (pink porcelain), because this affects the extent of preprosthetic surgery needed. The early involvement of the ceramist in every procedure also relates to managing patient expectations, because a thorough discussion between dentist and ceramist allows the dentist to explain any limitations of a procedure to the patient at the beginning.

INITIAL RECORDS
Photography

The dentist-ceramist team relies heavily on the use of photography, a topic covered in depth elsewhere in this issue. Essentially, the clinician moves through a series of facial (face and teeth), dental-facial (lips and teeth), and dental photographs (teeth only) (**Fig. 1**). These photographs, beginning with the full face and zooming in to analyze just the teeth, help the team move through a mental checklist of diagnostic criteria, from macroesthetic to microesthetic elements. The macroesthetic elements are those such as midline canting, incisal plane, and buccal corridor, whereas the microesthetic

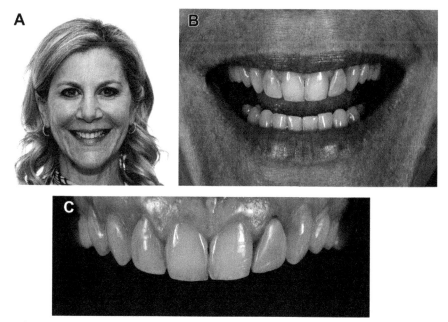

Fig. 1. The facial, dental-facial, and dental perspectives. (*A*) Face and teeth. (*B*) Lips and teeth. (*C*) Teeth only.

elements include aspects such as zenith levels, axial inclinations, and shade.[2] These facial, dental-facial, and dental photographs will be repeated after the provisionals are cemented, and again on cementation of the final restorations. **Table 1** shows the complete list of macroesthetic and microesthetic elements that are analyzed as these photographs are taken.

In our offices, we have recently also incorporated video, allowing us to more fully grasp our patients' wants and needs by seeing who they are and what they want to gain from this experience. From a diagnostic perspective, video allows us to capture each patient's lip dynamics during speaking, and phonetic analysis, both of which are hard to capture via still photography alone. Technically, the simple setup consists of a

Table 1		
Macroesthetic and microesthetic elements to analyze while taking photographs		
Facial (Macroesthetic)	**Dental-Facial (Macroesthetic)**	**Dental (Microesthetic)**
• Interpupillary line to occlusal plane • Dental midline to facial midline • Nasolabial angle • Ricketts e-plane • Dominant/nondominant sides + facial symmetry	• Height of smile • Tooth exposure at rest • Dental midline to philtrum • Degree of buccal corridor • Amount of teeth displayed in smile	• Tooth form • Tooth proportions • Shade • Axial inclinations • Zenith positions • Papilla positions • Embrasures and contacts • Texture • Translucency • Opalescence

tripod-mounted 4K high-definition (HD) video camera with a light-emitting diode (LED) ring light (**Fig. 2**). The patients are seated in front of a black backdrop and asked to discuss their expectations, then asked to smile both naturally and with an exaggerated smile. A video of no longer than 30 seconds should be sufficient, and, from this video, HD still images can be extracted for analysis.

Kois Dento-Facial Analyzer

The maxillary and mandibular impressions obtained at the initial appointment, either conventionally with polyvinyl siloxane (PVS) or via intraoral scan, must be related to the true horizontal plane before any esthetic improvements can be made. To accomplish this, we use the Kois dento-facial analyzer, a replacement for the conventional ear-borne facebow. It is well known that the ears (and all facial features) are more often than not asymmetrical.[3] The Kois dento-facial analyzer is essentially a fox plane, with leveling bubbles and a perpendicular vertical post meant to represent the midline (**Fig. 3**). This device allows us to orient the maxillary plane in relation to the true horizon, instead of relying on facial features. The mounting plate is transferred to an articulator at a set 100-mm axis-incisal distance. According to Dr Jon Kois' research, "approximately 80% of the population are within 5 mm of the average 100 mm axis-incisal distance, which is approximately the same percentage reported in research comparing arbitrary earbows."[4] In the authors' experience, even large-scale cases involving occlusal vertical dimension change can be successfully performed using this system in lieu of a traditional facebow. Once the maxillary cast is mounted, the mandibular cast can be mounted against it, using a PVS bite registration material, or, whenever possible, hand articulation. The mounted models, together with the

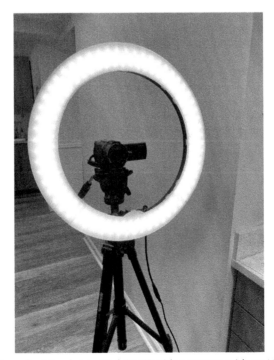

Fig. 2. Simple setup of a tripod-mounted 4K-HD video camera with an LED ring light.

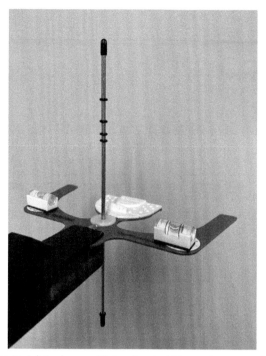

Fig. 3. A Kois Dento-Facial Analyzer, with leveling bubbles and a perpendicular vertical post meant to represent the midline.

complete diagnostic photographic series, allow a diagnostic wax-up that allows us to evaluate the function and esthetics of our proposed smile design.

Ideal Maxillary Central Incisor Length and Incisal Plane

There are many ways to convey the esthetic plan to the ceramist, but, at the minimum, the clinician must determine at the initial records visit (1) the ideal maxillary central incisor edge position as it relates to the face, and (2) the true horizon, which is also the incisal plane. Having these 2 references, combined with the diagnostic photographs, allows the ceramist to design the entire smile, following the many well-known rules of esthetics.[5] Assuming the existing incisal edge position is not acceptable (sometimes it is), the authoring team's 3 most common methods for visualizing the ideal central incisor position are:

- Chairside flowable composite (**Fig. 4**) can be added to deficient maxillary central incisal edges quickly and easily. This composite can be reduced with a sandpaper disk if needed, until it looks appropriately long and appropriately level with the horizon. Once established, an impression or intraoral scan of the arch is taken, to be used for a waxing index. The flowable composite can be added to just the 2 central incisors, or (even more helpful for the ceramist) extended to the anterior 6 or 8 teeth. Two photographs of the entire face, smiling with teeth apart and with lips separated at rest, are also taken at this point (**Fig. 5**) to confirm our placement of the maxillary central incisal edge.
- Black Sharpie: if a tooth is too long and the solution might be to shorten it, a black Sharpie is used to simulate the reduced tooth length (**Fig. 6**). This

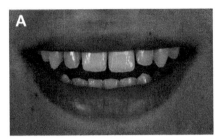
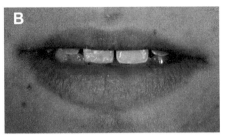

Fig. 4. Chairside flowable composite added to tooth #8 to match the length of #9.

simulation could then be photographed alongside a periodontal probe for measurement.

- Digital planning. By laying a grid over the face, we can establish vertical and horizontal references, plan the ideal tooth positions based on the face, and then calibrate the design to real-world measurements. Two examples of digital planning protocols are Photoshop Smile Design (Ed McLaren) and Digital Smile Design (Christian Coachman).[6]

Detailed Laboratory Prescription

This prescription is a written description giving as much detail as possible and identifying the patient's goals. **Fig. 7** gives an example of a typical laboratory prescription. Remember it is the clinician's responsibility to convey the patient's hopes and expectations to the ceramist accurately.

The following list shows the items that must go to the ceramist after the first appointment, in order to obtain an ideal functional and esthetic wax-up:

- Maxillary and mandibular impressions or scans
- Bite registration (either PVS or scan) in maximum intercuspation or centric relation depending on the procedure
- Kois mounting plate
- Impression/scan of proposed ideal maxillary incisal edge or digital design
- Complete set of diagnostic photographs

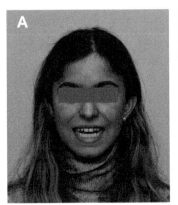
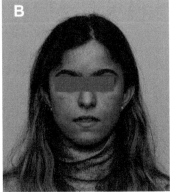

Fig. 5. (A) The entire face, smiling with teeth apart. (B) The entire face, with lips separated at rest.

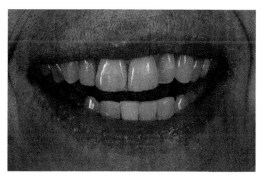

Fig. 6. If a tooth is too long and the solution might be to shorten it, a black marker is used to simulate the reduced tooth length.

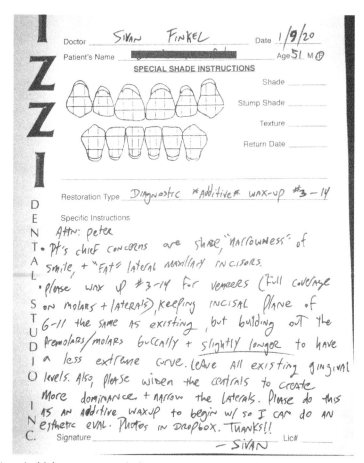

Fig. 7. A typical laboratory prescription.

- Laboratory prescription

All these records drive the diagnostic wax-up. When the wax-up is completed, the patient returns for the crucial second step in the process: the esthetic evaluation.

DIAGNOSTIC WAX-UP AND ESTHETIC EVALUATION

It is critically important to show the patient what we are planning, before picking up a handpiece and irreversibly altering the teeth. To achieve this, whenever the situation permits, we test our design intraorally and in the context of the face and lips. This step, the esthetic evaluation, is an opportunity not only for the patient to visualize the proposed treatment but also for the clinician-ceramist team to confirm that the design makes functional and esthetic sense.

The records described earlier drive our wax-up (**Fig. 8**), which becomes the blueprint to the procedure. It is worth noting that the author charges a fee for the diagnostic wax-up, and explains to the patient that it will:

1. Allow the patient to visualize the outcome
2. Become the template for the provisionals (temporaries)
3. Help us keep the amount of tooth preparation as minimal as possible

A wax-up can either be done additively, with no reduction performed on the stone model, or reductively, where the stone model is modified first to make the wax-up more ideal. Examples of additive wax-ups include diastema closure, or cases where purely length and volume are added to the teeth. Examples of reductive wax-ups include midline correction, or cases that involve shortening teeth or reducing tooth mass. Making the distinction between additive and reductive is important, because only additive wax-ups can be transferred into the mouth without any tooth reduction. Because the esthetic evaluation step is so critical, in patients requiring reduction, the ceramist produces 2 wax-ups: a less ideal, additive-only version, for the purpose of esthetic evaluation and patient motivation, and an ideal reductive version, for the purpose of provisionals and preparation control. In cases where we are shortening incisal edges or cusps, the additive wax-up shows the original stone projecting beyond the wax, and this area is blacked out with a fine Sharpie once the wax-up is transferred to the mouth.

The wax-up is transferred to the mouth via an acrylic or putty index, using a bis-acryl material (**Fig. 9**). With the design in place, once again a video is taken of the patient speaking. The patients are encouraged to speak naturally and tell a story, but to keep their lips animated.

At this point, the patients should be shown the video of themselves, or selected screenshots from it. It is worth noting that, up until this point, the patient has not been given a handheld mirror. This bis-acryl design over unprepared teeth often does not look as beautiful as the provisionals and final porcelain will be, and patients could get discouraged or confused, especially in reductive cases when the

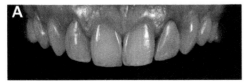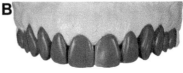

Fig. 8. A wax-up.

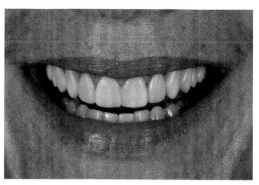

Fig. 9. The wax-up is transferred to the mouth via an acrylic or putty index, using a bis-acryl material.

purely additive first wax-up is noticeably bulkier than the second, ideal wax-up. For the patients, seeing the design for the first time through our video, from a conversational distance and in the context of their full faces (**Fig. 10**) is extremely impactful and helps motivate them to accept treatment. Still photographs can be extracted from the video and emailed to the patients if they would like some time to decide.

TOOTH PREPARATION

Just as the diagnostic wax-up communicates the esthetic vision to the patient, it is also the blueprint for the tooth preparation and thus an important communication tool between dentist and ceramist. The teeth should always be prepared in relation to the final volume and final position that the wax-up dictates, and according to the requirements of the specific material being preparing for. Putty indexes can be trimmed into buccal and incisal reduction guides, and an even more precise method is to prepare the teeth directly through the intraoral bis-acryl prototype. This method is known as the Aesthetic Pre-Evaluative Temporaries technique, first described by Galip Gurel.[7]

Once tooth preparation is completed (**Fig. 11**), impressions of the teeth are made conventionally or with an intraoral scanner. These are the full list of records that are sent to the laboratory at the completion of this appointment:

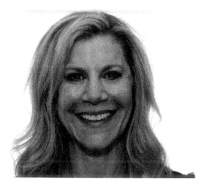

Fig. 10. For the patient, seeing the design from a conversational distance and in the context of the full face, is extremely impactful and helps motivate the patient to accept treatment.

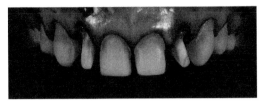

Fig. 11. Completed tooth preparations.

1. Final impression/scan of prepared teeth
2. Impression/scan of opposing arch
3. Bite registration; preps against lower arch, or prep to prep in full-mouth cases
4. Photographs
   a. Desired shade photographs: photographs, with shade tabs, of the relevant tooth/teeth being matched to.
   b. Preparation shade photos: photographs, with shade tabs, of the completed preparations. These photographs are usually taken with the teeth slightly moistened.
5. Diagnostic wax-up or impression/scan of provisionals if anything has been changed
6. Facial, dental-facial, and dental photographs of approved provisionals

PROVISIONALIZATION

Another powerful communication tool between the dental team and the patient is the provisionals (**Fig. 12**). Our provisionals allow the patients to test the shade and form of

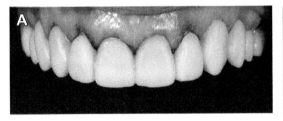
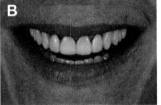
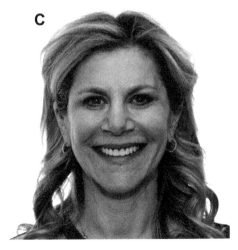

Fig. 12. Provisionals.

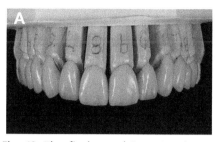
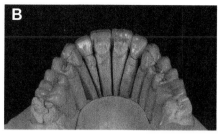

Fig. 13. The final porcelain restorations, a combination of laminate veneers and full coverage.

the final restorations, and the dental team should welcome any and all input. The patients are encouraged to be critical. In most cases, the patient is brought back a week later, without anesthesia and thus with regular lip mobility, to discuss the shade and form. Any changes to form are made chairside, photographs are retaken, and a new impression/scan is obtained for the ceramist.

TRY-IN AND CEMENTATION

Once the restorations are delivered to the clinician (**Fig. 13**), the patient returns and the provisionals are removed. The restorations are tried in, 1 by 1 and then all together. The restorations are usually tried in with just water, but, in the rare instance that the shade needs to be adjusted, colored try-in paste (followed by the corresponding colored cement) may be used.

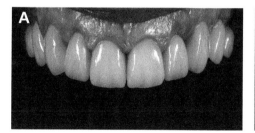
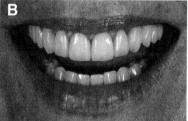

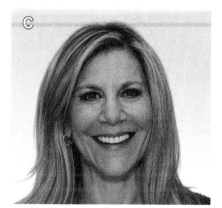

Fig. 14. Final photos.

The patient is shown the restorations seated without any cement, and, if approved, the restorations are cemented. Note that, before cementation during the try-in, (1) function cannot be tested, and (2) the patient does not have a chance to see these final restorations in the context of the entire face, only close-up and usually with the lips retracted. Phonetics cannot be tested with uncemented restorations either. It is for these reasons that it is imperative the final restorations follow the exact length of the approved provisionals.

FINAL FOLLOW-UP PHOTOGRAPHS

Two weeks following cementation, the patient returns for a follow-up visit, at which point we make any corrections to the occlusion, deliver a nightguard if necessary, and obtain our final photographs (**Fig. 14**). These final photographs are extremely important: even though the procedure is completed, the follow-up photographs allow us to self-evaluate, judge our work, and consider what we can improve next time.

In summary, thoughtful and thorough communication protocols between dentist, ceramist, and patient are critical to our success, especially in the realm of esthetics, where there is no right or wrong. The quality of our communication defines our ability to deliver the results that we promise.

DISCLOSURE

The authors have nothing to disclose.

REFERENCES

1. Coachman C, Gurel G, Calamita M, et al. The influence of tooth color on preparation design for laminate veneers from a minimally invasive perspective: case report. Int J Periodontics Restorative Dent 2014;34(4):453–9.
2. Levine JB, Finkel S. Chapter 1 - Esthetic diagnosis: a three-step analysis. In: Levine JB, editor. Essentials of esthetic dentistry: smile design integrating esthetics and function. New York: Elsevier; 2016. p. 1–42.
3. Namano S, Behrend DA, Harcourt JK, et al. Angular asymmetries of the human face. Int J Prosthodont 2000;13(1):41–6.
4. Tak On T, Kois JC. Digital smile design meets the dento-facial analyzer: optimizing esthetics while preserving tooth structure. Compend Contin Educ Dent 2016;37(1): 46–50.
5. Rufenacht CR. Fundamentals of esthetics. Hanover Park (IL): Quintessence; 1990. p. 116–9.
6. Coachman C, Calamita MA. Digital smile design: a tool for treatment planning and communication in esthetic dentistry. Quintessence Dent Technol 2012;35:103–11.
7. Gurel G. The science and art of porcelain laminate veneers. Chicago: Quintessence; 2003. p. 248, 249, 257, 260, 261, 485.

A Communication Guide for Orthodontic-Restorative Collaborations

An Orthodontic Perspective on the Importance of Working in a Team

Kathryn Preston, DDS, MS

KEYWORDS

- Orthodontic terminology • Orthodontic-restorative communication
- Orthodontic anterior esthetics • Smile esthetics • Occlusion

KEY POINTS

- Excellent communication between provider and patient, as well as between providers, is critical for case success.
- The restorative dentist's understanding of basic orthodontic terminology and general orthodontic case considerations is useful in optimizing communication.
- Although esthetics are an important component, the functional and biologic limitations of the hard and soft tissues need to be carefully respected.
- Though orthodontists use cephalometrics and normative data, these are just some of the considerations when developing their treatment plans and goals.
- Early and consistent involvement of both restorative dentists and specialists can help provide patients with more complete and informed decision-making abilities, and can improve outcomes.

INTRODUCTION: NATURE OF THE PROBLEM

Multidisciplinary cases can be some of our most challenging yet rewarding experiences as providers. Restorative and orthodontic collaborations are frequently encountered when discussing multidisciplinary care. It is not uncommon for restorative cases to benefit from some degree of orthodontic care to support an esthetic and functional result. Likewise, orthodontic cases often are esthetically improved by involving the restorative dentist in optimizing tooth morphology.

Section of Orthodontics, UCLA School of Dentistry, 10833 Le Conte Avenue, Box 951668, Los Angeles, CA 90095, USA
E-mail address: kpreston@dentistry.ucla.edu

Dent Clin N Am 64 (2020) 709–718
https://doi.org/10.1016/j.cden.2020.06.001
0011-8532/20/© 2020 Elsevier Inc. All rights reserved.

dental.theclinics.com

Communication is of paramount importance to a successful treatment outcome. Understanding the goals of our patients assists in managing and meeting their expectations. In multidisciplinary cases, excellent communication not only between provider and patient is expected, but seamless collaboration between the involved practitioners is a requirement in achieving an outcome of the highest standard. Similarly, patients should not only be fully participatory in treatment discussions, but they should be provided consultation with indicated specialists when appropriate. Communication at all levels is at the core of these concepts.

Logistical challenges are not uncommon, but at the heart of interprovider communication is using standard terminology. In this article, an introduction to basic orthodontic terminology often used to describe certain components of occlusion, function, and esthetics is presented. In addition, global insight into some comprehensive orthodontic case planning considerations will be discussed to indicate that it is more than just simple tooth positioning; rather, specialty knowledge is imperative in recognizing limitations of jaw relationships, as well as anticipated effects on the hard and soft tissues. The scope of this article is limited in nature to give the restorative dentist an introduction to several factors included in case assessment from an orthodontic perspective. It is intended to augment their awareness of orthodontic considerations, promote discussion among different specialties, and to encourage inclusion of multidisciplinary practitioners in case planning.

ASSESS THE PATIENT'S GOALS, AND BUILD YOUR TEAM

In the dental profession, we are gifted in that we have the ability to collaborate with both our patients and other colleagues in a concerted effort to achieve excellent results.

As illustrated in **Box 1**, first and foremost, it is important to ascertain the specific goals of the patient to determine what is and what is not in the realm of possibility with restorative and/or orthodontic treatment alone. Second, as the professional, it is our duty to determine if these esthetic goals are still supportive of overall function and health. Third, both specialists and restorative dentists must recognize when certain aspects of care are outside their realm of expertise, and must refer and consult accordingly. These concepts are in support of the American Dental Association's Code of Ethics and Professional Conduct, which highlights the importance of enabling patients to make fully informed treatment decisions, as well as providers recognizing the potential limitations in their own expertise.[1]

Of note, a patient's concern may not be able to be addressed by orthodontics or restorative means alone. An example of this might be a patient's discontent with a gummy smile, and the diagnosis may be vertical maxillary excess of a skeletal nature. Similarly, a patient may want to address a large overjet, but it is determined that the

---

Box 1
Questions to consider when evaluating a case

- What are the patient's expectations and goals?
- Is this goal achievable with restorative and/or orthodontic treatment alone?
- Can this esthetic goal be met while still providing an outcome that is functionally and periodontally sound?
- Do I have the knowledge base to make these multidisciplinary decisions? With which specialists do I need to confer?

skeletal discrepancy between the jaws is beyond simple tooth repositioning or restorative care. In these examples and others, certain presentations may benefit from surgical assistance to avoid jeopardizing oral health and function. Therefore, a third provider should be consulted, which is in many cases an oral and maxillofacial surgeon, to fully diagnose and triage certain cases as well. Although the emphasis in this article is on orthodontic and restorative communications, it should be noted that certain cases often require involvement of additional specialist providers to support case success as well.

In summary, it is recommended to involve the indicated specialists in the discussion and decision-making as early in the assessment process as possible. When referring to a specialist or any outside provider, creating a supportive document to indicate your findings and goals for the referral would also prove helpful. This team perspective of involving multiple qualified providers can work to provide the best comprehensive plan for our patients, and allow them to make more fully informed decisions.

GENERAL ORTHODONTIC TERMINOLOGY: THE BASICS OF COMMUNICATION

Initial orthodontic assessment of facial morphology and proportion is performed in 3 dimensions (anterior-posterior, transverse, and vertical) at rest and various active states, such as when smiling and speaking. Supplemental angles and views of the face also can be helpful. This evaluation is executed with clinical observation of the patient, as well as review of records in the form of photographs, radiographs, and study models. In the facial assessment, the entirety of the face is considered when developing an orthodontic treatment plan, but for the limited nature of this article, the focus is on the lower third.

The main ingredient to proper communication is standardizing terminology. No matter what terminology a dental team uses, it is critical to ensure it is consistent and there is full understanding of the definitions. Although not intended to be a comprehensive list of factors or considerations in orthodontic functional and esthetic assessment, this summary of basic terms (**Table 1**) may often be discussed when reviewing cases and should serve as an introduction to orthodontic terminology.

COMPREHENSIVE ORTHODONTIC CASE ASSESSMENT: CONSIDERATIONS BEYOND THE NUMBERS

Another important factor known to orthodontic specialists is the role of normative values in case assessment. What restorative dentists may not realize is that although specialists take these values into account, they do not necessarily let them dictate treatment absolutely. Although it is important for the restorative dentist to have an awareness of these concepts, a specialist should have the training and experience to understand the nuanced applications of these considerations at a higher level and can apply them to the decision-making process.

The normative and/or ideal values presented in the previous **Table 1**, as well as in other published literature regarding cephalometrics, imply that there are strict and narrow parameters for what is considered "esthetic"; this is simply not the case. Beauty truly is in the eye of the beholder and can vary immensely. A critical consideration to bear in mind when reviewing published hard and soft tissue normative values is that these often are population-specific, and norms and even esthetic preferences naturally vary between people of different ages, sexes, and ethnicities.[16,17] For instance, it is known that people of different ages, sexes, and ethnicities have varying soft tissue

Table 1
Basic orthodontic terminology in anterior esthetics

Term	Definition	Related General Esthetic Considerations
Overjet (Fig. 1)	Horizontal (anterior-posterior) distance measured from the labial surface of the mandibular incisors to the incisal edge of the maxillary incisors. • + value, if the maxillary anterior teeth are forward of the mandibular incisors. • − value, if the maxillary anterior teeth are posterior to the mandibular incisors (i.e., anterior crossbite)	The ideal is commonly +2 mm. Reverse overjet (in anterior crossbite) as well as significant excess overjet have been reported to be considered less esthetic.[2,3]
Overbite (Fig. 2)	Vertical overlap of the maxillary and mandibular anterior teeth. • + value, if the teeth overlap. • − value, if there is no vertical overlap of the anterior teeth (i.e., open bite)	The ideal is generally +2 mm. A deeper bite is more esthetically pleasing than an open bite, however.[4,5]
Smile arc (Fig. 3)	Relationship of the lower lip curvature with the arc formed by the incisal edges of the maxillary anterior teeth. • Described as reverse, flat, consonant, or excessive.	The maxillary incisal edges should follow the contour of the lower lip when smiling.[6] Consonant smile arcs are generally more preferred.[7,8]
Dental midlines (Fig. 4)	Midlines are generally taken between the maxillary and mandibular central incisors, and measured relative to one another as well as the facial midline.	Despite some variation in the literature, generally slight midline deviation (approximately 2–3 mm) may be considered acceptable, depending on the observer; however, angulated dental midlines (reportedly 10[°,9] or 2 mm as measured from papilla to incisal embrasure[10]) tend to be more noticeable and less desirable, as discussed in a systematic review.[11]
Buccal corridors (Fig. 5)	Space observed between the buccal surfaces of the maxillary posterior teeth and the inside of the cheeks when smiling. This may impact the appearance or perception of a full or narrow smile.	Based on review of studies assessing natural smile images rather than digitally induced buccal corridors, the presence of buccal corridors does not necessarily detract from smile esthetics.[11] The literature is inconsistent with regard to acceptable buccal corridor dimensions.[8]

Occlusal canting	Asymmetric tilting of the occlusion, when viewed from the frontal perspective.	Generally, the line following the incisal edges of the anterior teeth should be parallel to the interpupillary line (assuming level orbits), and therefore no occlusal canting.[12,13] An occlusal cant has been reported to be observed when exceeding 2.8°,[4] or when the incisal plane is rotated 1–3 mm.[10]
Gingival display (**Fig. 6**, in green)	Vertical assessment of maxillary gingiva observed when smiling.	This varies depending on age and sex, with younger female individuals tending to have more gingival reveal than older male individuals. With regard to esthetic preference, the literature is variable on indicating the threshold for acceptability.[8]
Incisal display (see **Fig. 6**, in red)	Vertical assessment of maxillary incisor show while at rest and when smiling.	This varies depending on age and sex, with younger female individuals tending to have more incisal display than older male individuals.[6,14] Like gingival display, the esthetic parameters and etiology of incisal display are multifactorial.[15]

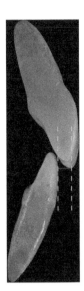

Fig. 1. Overjet (in *red*).

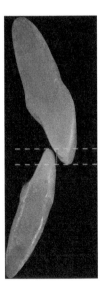

Fig. 2. Overbite (in *red*).

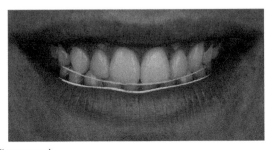

Fig. 3. Smile arc (in *orange*).

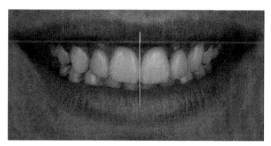

Fig. 4. Dental midlines (in *orange*).

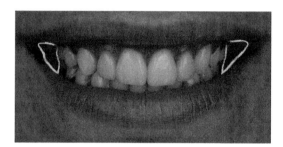

Fig. 5. Buccal corridors (in *blue*).

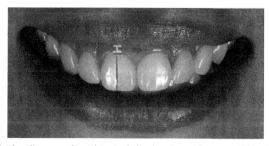

Fig. 6. Gingival display (in *green*) and incisal display (in *red*), on smiling. At rest not shown.

thicknesses, and therefore often respond to treatment differently; this individuality can impact treatment goals and the mechanics needed to achieve them.

Likewise, although numerical normative values can be useful, they do not necessarily ensure a clinically esthetic outcome.[18,19] Rather, these values should be treated more as guidelines and not necessarily as mandatory treatment goals in every case. Similarly, an advanced understanding of these values includes knowing the related factors that can impact them, and accounting for that in the treatment decision-making process. In orthodontics, we often say "don't treat to the numbers," and this mantra implies this principle: aim to treat to a facial and occlusal esthetic outcome that still provides oral health and functional stability, and not solely to satisfy cephalometric or anthropometric normative data. In other words, an esthetic outcome that is still simultaneously supportive of health and function may not necessarily always reflect agreement with hard and soft tissue normative values. Each case should be considered independently, and objectives set accordingly; orthodontic care is not a one-size-fits-all service.

Orthognathic surgery literature discusses similar philosophies of treating to esthetic visual proportions in their field, rather than absolute quantitative normalcy.[20,21] Surgeons, like other specialists, are trained to combine the art and science of their discipline to maximize facial balance and harmony while planning for stable and healthy results. However, it should be emphasized that overriding the normative values does not give permission for full subjectivity without regard for the biologic limitations of the occlusion, periodontium, or facial structures. Rather, intelligently and prudently weighing the visual qualitative assessment with the numerical quantitative measurements in the context of the entire patient presentation is an important skill needed in comprehensive case planning. As always, the biologic limitations should be respected.

With software options and appliances on the market that offer diagnosis assistance, case planning support, and appliance fabrication, technology can aid the provider in making and carrying out treatment decisions. However, a limited understanding of specialty principles, including those presented here, might mistakenly lead some providers to believe that these systems or appliances can accurately deliver specialist-level results, often in place of the case itself being assessed by a specialist. It is important to recognize that these systems are tools to be wielded wisely with proper education and with full understanding that, despite advances in technology, they are not substitutes for good clinical judgment and experience.

In summary, it is important to evaluate cases on their own merit and with comprehensive team expertise. Software should be used to aid providers, and not substitute for them. Blindly following numerical norms or not recognizing unique age, sex, and ethnicity factors can hinder case success. Recognizing the unique considerations of each case provides a more global, advanced understanding of the complexities involved in excellent care, and the indicated specialists should be sought out to provide this knowledge in multidisciplinary cases.

SUMMARY

Team care is of benefit to the patient and all providers involved in the case. It is important to recognize that restorative dentists and specialists all have their respective areas of expertise, and should be consulted accordingly on multidisciplinary cases. It is not the job of the restorative dentist to personally fulfill every role on the team, and therefore they are expected to recruit specialist teammates to support excellent and comprehensive care. The goal of this article is to encourage the dialogue of trained and experienced specialists and restorative dentists with one another and with patients to devise esthetic outcomes that are supportive of overall oral health and function, using the unique skills of each provider in unison rather than in place of the other.

This pursuit of excellence starts with unifying terminology to achieve effective communication of goals, expectations, and limitations. In addition, a deeper comprehension of normative values and their role in treatment planning is important for a more complete understanding of case assessment. Furthermore, effective treatment is not simply treating to what a cephalometric or software program dictates, but rather to use excellent clinical training and sound judgment to help ensure an esthetic and functional outcome; this goal can more readily be achieved through involvement and proper communication within a skilled and knowledgeable team.

DISCLOSURE

The author has nothing to disclose.

REFERENCES

1. American Dental Association. Principles of Ethics and Code of Professional Conduct. 2018. Available at: https://www.ada.org/~/media/ADA/Member%20Center/Ethics/Code_Of_Ethics_Book_With_Advisory_Opinions_Revised_to_November_2018.pdf?la=en. Accessed January 30, 2020.
2. Soh J, Chew MT, Chan YH. Perceptions of dental esthetics of Asian orthodontists and laypersons. Am J Orthod Dentofac Orthop 2006;130(2):170–6.
3. Sierwald I, John MT, Schierz O, et al. Association of overjet and overbite with esthetic impairments of oral health-related quality of life. J Orofac Orthop 2015; 76(5):405–20.
4. Springer NC, Chang C, Fields HW, et al. Smile esthetics from the layperson's perspective. Am J Orthod Dentofac Orthop 2011;139(1):e91–101.
5. Chang CA, Fields HW Jr, Beck FM, et al. Smile esthetics from patients' perspectives for faces of varying attractiveness. Am J Orthod Dentofac Orthop 2011; 140(4):e171–80.
6. Sarver DM. The importance of incisor positioning in the esthetic smile: the smile arc. Am J Orthod Dentofac Orthop 2001;120(2):98–111.
7. Parekh S, Fields HW, Beck FM, et al. The acceptability of variations in smile arc and buccal corridor space. Orthod Craniofac Res 2007;10(1):15–21.
8. Parrini S, Rossini G, Castroflorio T, et al. Laypeople's perceptions of frontal smile esthetics: a systematic review. Am J Orthod Dentofac Orthop 2016;150(5): 740–50.
9. Thomas JL, Hayes C, Zawaideh S. The effect of axial midline angulation on dental esthetics. Angle Orthod 2003;73(4):359–64.
10. Kokich VO Jr, Kiyak HA, Shapiro PA. Comparing the perception of dentists and lay people to altered dental esthetics. J Esthet Dent 1999;11(6):311–24.
11. Janson G, Branco NC, Fernandes TMF, et al. Influence of orthodontic treatment, midline position, buccal corridor and smile arc on smile attractiveness. Angle Orthod 2011;81(1):153–61.
12. Sharma PK, Sharma P. Dental smile esthetics: the assessment and creation of the ideal smile. Semin Orthod 2012;18(3):193–201.
13. Reyneke JP, Ferretti C. Clinical assessment of the face. Semin Orthod 2012;18(3): 172–86.

14. Fudalej P. Long-term changes of the upper lip position relative to the incisal edge. Am J Orthod Dentofac Orthop 2008;133(2):204–9.
15. Desai S, Upadhyay M, Nanda R. Dynamic smile analysis: changes with age. Am J Orthod Dentofac Orthop 2009;136(3):310.e1-10.
16. Hall D, Taylor RW, Jacobson A, et al. The perception of optimal profile in African Americans versus white Americans as assessed by orthodontists and the lay public. Am J Orthod Dentofac Orthop 2000;118(5):514–25.
17. Vela E, Taylor RW, Campbell PM, et al. Differences in craniofacial and dental characteristics of adolescent Mexican Americans and European Americans. Am J Orthod Dentofac Orthop 2011;140(6):839–47.
18. Sarver DM, Ackerman JL. Orthodontics about face: The re-emergence of the esthetic paradigm. Am J Orthod Dentofac Orthop 2000;117(5):575–6.
19. Nanda RS, Ghosh J. Facial soft tissue harmony and growth in orthodontic treatment. Semin Orthod 1995;1(2):67–81.
20. Rosen HM. Evolution of a surgical philosophy in orthognathic surgery. Plast Reconstr Surg 2017;139(4):978–90.
21. Selber JC, Rosen HM. Aesthetics of facial skeletal surgery. Clin Plast Surg 2007; 34(3):437–45.

A Communication Guide for Orthodontic-Restorative Collaborations

Digital Smile Design Outline Tool

Yair Y. Whiteman, DMD

KEYWORDS

- Multidisciplinary • Restorative • Orthodontics • Communication
- Digitally-driven smile design outline tool

KEY POINTS

- Orthodontic-restorative multidisciplinary collaboration is a critical aspect in esthetic and functional treatment outcome.
- Ideally, orthodontic-restorative cases are planned jointly.
- Facially driven esthetic evaluation sequence is imperative for structured and organized treatment planning, and the digital outline tool is used to streamline the team's communication, which can support orthodontic-restorative improved treatment outcome.

INTRODUCTION

Whenever orthodontic-restorative treatments are performed, it is essential to comprehensively assess the case, establish treatment objectives, and plan the sequence and execution of the interdisciplinary treatment in advance of starting any procedure.[1–3] Not including all providers early in the treatment planning process can potentially increase overall treatment time, as well as be burdensome for the patient if changes need to be made unexpectedly due to lack of communication. For instance, the restorative dentist may be put in the position of restoring the dentition with compromised spacing and clearance when simple communication between providers could have prevented this concern. Alternatively, if a dentist proceeds with placing restorations before the patient initiates orthodontic treatment, the occlusion may change and merit costly restorative replacement and additional treatment.

Communication and progress follow-up are critical when seeking ideal outcome. One additional challenge in the orthodontic-restorative collaborative case

Division of Constitutive and Regenerative Science, UCLA School of Dentistry, 10833 Le-Conte Avenue, Room 33-064A CHS, Los Angeles, CA 90095-1668, USA
E-mail address: ywhiteman@dentistry.ucla.edu

Dent Clin N Am 64 (2020) 719–730
https://doi.org/10.1016/j.cden.2020.06.002
0011-8532/20/© 2020 Elsevier Inc. All rights reserved.

management is the ability to evaluate case readiness for the completion of the ortho-dontic phase. Often in the final steps of the orthodontic treatment, the orthodontist will refer the patient for a restorative esthetic evaluation and verification before removing the orthodontic appliances. At this point, the restoring dentist will often be asked to determine if the position of the teeth is appropriate for completion of the orthodontic phase and initiating of the restorative phase of the treatment. This article discusses a workflow that can streamline the team's ability to establish treatment strategies, eval-uate progress, and effectively communicate course of action when needed.

CONSIDERATIONS FOR MULTIDISCIPLINARY TEAM MEMBERS

The multidisciplinary patient care approach has been shown to be undeniably advan-tageous for patients as well as providers. The ability to include a number of qualified providers with specific skill sets while developing a coordinated treatment strategy en-ables us a far more controlled treatment environment and ultimately improved outcome.[4] To support the excellence of the team, members should continue to educate themselves as treatment protocols evolve as well as strive to maintain excel-lent communication. Likewise, it is important to share similar evidence-based treat-ment philosophies to support treatment decisions.

From the restorative dentist's perspective, it is essential that the orthodontist in the team will know what the restorative possibilities are, understand material limitations and space requirements, and develop an ability to visualize proper tooth position to accept restorations once the orthodontic treatment has been completed.[5–7] Just as orthodontists should have awareness of restorative concepts, restorative dentists must also have a respect and appreciation for orthodontic concepts, which includes fundamental biologic limitations of the periodontium with regard to tooth movement. Orthodontists also incorporate growth and development principles in their treatment planning, and can aid the restorative dentist in planning the timeline for definitive restorative care. Dentists must recognize how orthodontics can serve as a preparatory step before reductive restorative treatment is initiated, know fundamental orthodontic terminology, and be aware of biomechanics and other restrictions when planning a treatment.

COMMON ORTHODONTIC-RESTORATIVE CASES CRITICAL FOR CLOSE COORDINATION AND COMMUNICATION

The following is a general list of common interdisciplinary orthodontic-restorative cases encountered in our patient population.

1. Spacing and space management: crowding, diastema, hypodontia and partial edentulism, and microdontia (ie, peg laterals).[3,8,9]
2. Worn dentition: with or without loss of vertical dimension of occlusion (VDO).[9–11]
3. Position and realignment of teeth to allow more conservative tooth reduction for direct or indirect restorative treatment.
4. Gingival disharmony: excessive gingival display, disharmonious levels, as well as architecture and imperfect contours.[12,13]
5. Orthodontic extrusion to create a nonsurgical ferrule to restore root canal–treated teeth with post and core.[14]
6. Correction of occlusal plane and improved envelope of function.[9,13,15]
7. Reposition teeth to allow space for implant placement, implant site switching, and forced eruption to improve bone level.[13,16,17]

PURPOSE OF DIGITAL SMILE DESIGN TOOL IN ORTHODONTIC-RESTORATIVE COMMUNICATION

Ideally, the restorative dentist should have an opportunity to conduct his or her own assessment before placement of orthodontic appliances. Having these appliances in place makes it particularly challenging to visualize teeth positions, contours, and anatomy. Moreover, the gingiva is often hypertrophic due to inflammation during orthodontic treatment, and it is a suboptimal environment to acquire an impression for proper diagnostic evaluation. These are important considerations for planning a treatment that is, designed to optimize the overall facial and smile esthetics.

The beauty of applying facially driven smile design fundamentals[18–20] with basic digital smile design tools[21] (DSD) is that they can be used in case planning before or even during orthodontic appliance therapy, and therefore minimize much of the aforementioned concerns. The outline component of this tool is perhaps the most critical in optimizing near-immediate communication between providers and patients. This tool can help dentists and patients visualize possible outcome, communicate goals, and evaluate progress and ultimate readiness related to the esthetic outcome in orthodontic-restorative cases (**Fig. 1**).

The overall dentofacial evaluation sequence is outlined in **Box 1**. More detailed evaluation is described by the macro-esthetic and micro-esthetic evaluation, which is ultimately communicated using the DSD outline tool. Macro-esthetics and micro-

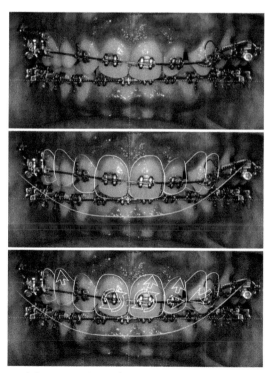

Fig. 1. DSD outline tool demonstrating esthetic evaluation of a case as presented on restorative examination. The tool also allows for visual communication back to the orthodontist to indicate recommended tooth movements to optimize the ultimate restorative outcome, as demonstrated by the white arrows in the third image.

Box 1
Dentofacial evaluation sequence checklist

1. Midline and horizontal lines
2. Identify maxillary incisal edge position
3. Establish and follow smile-line
4. Proper central incisor proportion
5. Interdental proportion
6. Teeth outline and arrangement
   a. Teeth general shape
   b. Smile line
   c. Incisal arrangement (flat, gal-wing)
7. Transfer outline to smile and full-face image.

---

esthetics will be evaluated once the teeth outline has been established later in the protocol. For the purpose of this article "macro-esthetics" refers to teeth relative to the patient's face and smile dynamics, whereas "micro-esthetics" refers to tooth shape and size, interdental and intradental proportions, as well as arrangement in the arch.[12,22]

Restorative dentists should assess the following macro-esthetic and micro-esthetic components to determine case progress and readiness for the restorative phase, as indicated in **Boxes 2** and **3**.

It is important to note, however, that certain limitations exist in using the DSD outline tool. Due to the 2-dimensional system, it might prevent evaluation of teeth proclination, overjet, open bite, malocclusion, plane of occlusion, and anterior-posterior (A-P) dimension relative to tooth display. Furthermore, because of photographic limitations,[23] we cannot rely on the digital outline alone and must also supplement with more precise measurements (ie, interbracket space distance, 3-dimensional scanning, impressions, and other measurement tools) in the assessment, particularly as the case is nearing completion of orthodontic treatment. Therefore, these detailed supplemental measurements must be evaluated before finalizing the orthodontic phase of treatment.[12,24,25]

PHOTOGRAPHS REQUIRED FOR DIGITAL SMILE DESIGN

At minimum, 5 images are required to produce a proper smile evaluation using the DSD tool, which ultimately all will serve to produce the final smile evaluation. These

---

Box 2
Macro-esthetic components to be evaluated in the digital smile design outline tool

1. Midlines
2. Smile line
3. Occlusal canting
4. Dentogingival interface
   a. Gingival display
   b. Gingival canting
   c. Gingival levels and harmony
   d. Gingival symmetry

Box 3
Micro-esthetics to be evaluated in the digital smile design outline tool

1. Individual tooth shape
2. Individual tooth size proportion (intradental)
3. Teeth proportions (interdental)
4. Teeth arrangement
5. Teeth axis and angulation
6. Dentogingival interface
   a. Gingival architecture
   b. scalloping
7. Overbite

---

photographs, when sequenced as described, can be considered as layers supportive of one another to collectively develop the smile esthetic evaluation on its own as well as in harmony with the face as whole. Additional images, videos, and patient feedback, as well as clinician observation and artistry can all be valuable in augmenting the esthetic assessment.[23,26,27]

These photographs should be uploaded and imported into the dentist's or technician's preferred software (Keynote, PowerPoint, or comparable smile design program can be used). The images (**Box 4**) are used as indicated in the following:

1. The portrait images (smile, retracted, lips at rest) aid in facially driven smile design evaluation. These involve full-face images that serve as initial orientation. Once close-up images are assessed, we return to the portrait images in the final step.
   i. The smile image is used to establish facial midline, horizontal lines, and smile line, as well as to evaluate gingival display.
   ii. The retracted portrait image allows visualization of the teeth in space without being obscured by surrounding facial soft tissue, and is used to evaluate horizontal cants.
   iii. Lips at rest image is used to evaluate incisal display; typically, 2.0 to 4.0 mm of incisor display at rest is considered esthetically favorable[18,28,29] and serves as our starting point for placing the maxillary incisal edge position.

Box 4
Required images for digital smile design to use the outline tool

1. Portrait (full face) view
   a. Full smile (maximum display)
   b. Retracted: teeth together in occlusion with retracted soft tissue
   c. Lips at rest (Repose)
2. Close-Up view
   a. Smile
   b. Retracted
3. Optional additional images
   a. Portrait + retracted: teeth apart
   b. 12 o'clock
   c. Profile
   d. Portrait and close-up side views

---

2. Close-up images of the dentition are acquired during smiling and lip retraction. The development of the smile design is performed on these images, before transferring back to the full-face portrait for final evaluation.

It is important to take all images in a uniform plane and orientation[23,27] such that patients are looking parallel to the horizon, as if they are looking at themselves in a mirror. In addition, the dentist or technician needs to calibrate the image sizes and crop them appropriately to scale before initiating the following protocol. This will help in workflow continuity and will aid in precision and reliability of the final product. This first step is important and provides the foundation on which we will develop the esthetic blueprint.

WORKFLOW FOR DIGITAL SMILE DESIGN OUTLINE TOOL

Once the dentist or technician has successfully acquired and imported the necessary photographs, a sequence is followed to perform the DSD evaluation. This section outlines the workflow.

To protect patient privacy, only close-up images are shown in this article. However, the steps including portrait images are still essential for a proper esthetic evaluation, and are described.

Step 1: Establish Facial Midline and Horizontal Lines

Using the Portrait images, facial midline is a vertical line generally found in the patient's midface.[20,21,30,31] It can be placed by visualizing the most suitable overall midpoint position in relation to the face, very similar to the midline generated during denture fabrication. Another method would be marking a center line between the patient's pupils perpendicular to the interpupillary line.

To mark the horizontal line, again use the patient's pupils as a reference point, and mark the center of the pupils and connect these points. In circumstances in which midline or interpupillary lines are not ideal due to facial or orbital asymmetry, select the most appropriate horizontal line by looking at the patient's overall full-facial images.

Once done, duplicate the horizontal line and position it in the projected maxillary incisal position in the Close-Up retracted image, as demonstrated in **Fig. 2**. It is recommended to place the incisal horizontal line close to the ideal estimated maxillary central incisal position based off of the image demonstrating lip at rest position, as it will help simplify workflow and evaluation process.

Both midline and horizontal lines are then moved to the Close-Up retracted image to establish virtual face-bow transfer. From this point on, most of the sequence will take place on the Close-Up retracted image and once completed, will be transferred to the Close-Up smile and Portrait smile images for further evaluation.

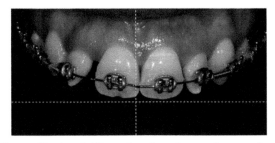

Fig. 2. Facial midline and horizontal lines placed on close-up images, demonstrating virtual face-bow transfer.

Step 2: Establish and Follow Smile Line

Using the patients' smile image (either Portrait or Close-Up), use the software's "shape tool" to follow and mark the lower lip line from oral commissure to the opposite corner to generate the smile line, as demonstrated in **Fig. 3**. Smile arc should follow the curvature of the lower lip.[31] Ideally, the smile arc of the incisal edges of the maxillary incisors and canines follows the smile line.[32] The smile line can now be transferred to the retracted Close-Up image, as shown in **Fig. 4**.

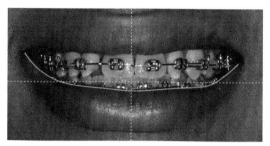

Fig. 3. Smile line (in *green*) parallels the curvature of the lower lip.

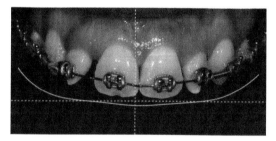

Fig. 4. Smile line is transferred to retracted close-up image.

Step 3: Tooth Proportion Tool

Average central maxillary incisors length to width ratio ranges from 70% to 85%[33]; however, the most esthetically acceptable range reported in the literature is 75% to 85%.[31] Consequently, depending on facial features and patient desire or as a starting point, a rectangular frame within this range is placed over one of the central incisors, as demonstrated in **Fig. 5**. Place the base of the frame on desired incisal position and

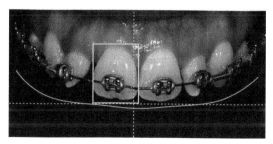

Fig. 5. Tooth proportion tool (*blue*) on retracted close-up image.

resize frame to desired size while keeping proportions constrained to maintain correct tooth ratio.

Step 4: Teeth Proportion Tool and Interdental Proportion

Different interdental proportion philosophies have been proposed and overridden in literature in the past decades.[30,34–37] In the University of California Los Angeles Center for Esthetic Dentistry (CED), the Recurring Esthetic Dental proportion (RED) tool is used as a starting point; however, golden proportions can also be used to evaluate symmetry, dominance, and interdental proportion.[35] It is important to remember that in the smile design process, using proportion tools serves as a starting point only and does not define the exact final ratios of the teeth.

Using a pre-made proportion guide, as shown in **Fig. 6**, resize the selected interdental proportion tool to fit previously placed central proportion frame and align it with the incisal position. It is important to maintain correct ratio when adjusting the size to maintain proper proportions.

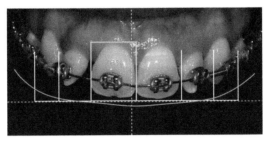

Fig. 6. Proportion ruler (*white*) is sized to fit preformed central proportion tool (*blue*). Both are placed on projected maxillary incisal edge.

Step 5: Teeth Outline and Arrangement

In this step, teeth outline is created by using existing downloaded libraries, outlining the patient's teeth, or by outlining other patients' teeth images. It is recommended to create a personal library from which the clinician or technician can pick and choose, thus being able to develop personalized smile designs for patients.

The teeth outline is then transferred and placed to fit into previously determined interdental proportion guidelines, as shown in **Fig. 7**. The teeth outline will now be resized to fit into the interdental proportion tool. At this point, the clinician can

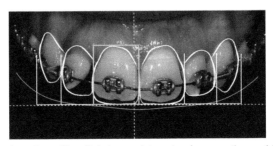

Fig. 7. Personalized teeth outline fit into predetermined proportion guidelines.

personalize and fine-tune the teeth outline, shape, and length, refine smile arc, and improve incisal design and gingival architecture to tailor to the patient's esthetic needs and wishes.

Step 6: Removal of Reference Lines and Proportion Tools

At this point, all auxiliary guide marks (facial midline and horizontal lines, as well as proportion tools) can be removed and evaluation for teeth position can take place. Only the teeth outline should remain (**Fig. 8**).

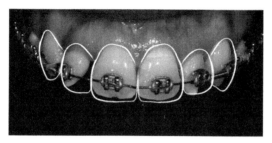

Fig. 8. Teeth outline on retracted view.

Step 7: Final Esthetic Evaluation

Once DSD steps are completed on the retracted Close-Up image, the teeth outline can now be transferred to smile images (both Close-Up and Portrait) for esthetic evaluation and communication with the patient and other team members, and case can move forward for completion. See **Figs. 9–12** for reference.

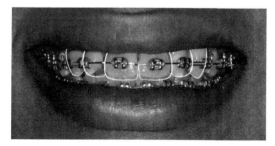

Fig. 9. Outline tool transferred to smile for evaluation.

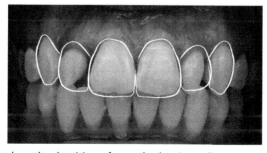

Fig. 10. Outline tool on the dentition after orthodontic appliance removal.

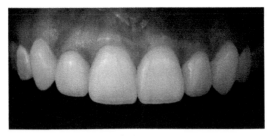

Fig. 11. Case completed close-up retracted view.

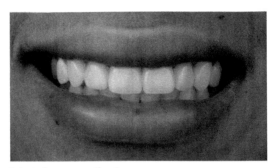

Fig. 12. Case completed close-up smile view.

SUMMARY

Orthodontic-restorative cases require precise communication before and during treatment. The challenge frequently met in many of these cases is finding a reliable and easy-to-interpret method for communicating goals and recommendations. The described visual benefits of the outline tool in the DSD technique can stream line the communication process and help ensure understanding among clinicians and patients.

ACKNOWLEDGMENT

Special thanks to Dr. Kanwar Singh-Sachdeva and Dr. Chirag Chawan from UCLA Orthodontics Postgraduate Program as well as Dr. Heba Binabid and Mr. Juan Kang from UCLA Center for Esthetic Dentistry for their involvement in the cases presented.

DISCLOSURE

The author has nothing to disclose.

REFERENCES

1. Kokich VG, Spear FM. Guidelines for managing the orthodontic-restorative patient. Semin Orthod 1997;3(1):3–20.
2. Spear FM, Kokich VG. A multidisciplinary approach to esthetic dentistry. Dent Clin North Am 2007;51(2):487–505, x-xi.
3. Gahan MJ, Lewis BR, Moore D, et al. The orthodontic-restorative interface: 1. Patient assessment. Dent Update 2010;37(2):74–6, 78-80.

4. Spear FM. Forming an interdisciplinary team: a key element in practicing with confidence and efficiency. J Am Dent Assoc 2005;136(10):1463–4.
5. McLaren EA, Whiteman YY. Ceramics: rationale for material selection. Compend Contin Educ Dent 2010;31(9):666–8, 670, 672 passim; quiz: 680, 700.
6. McLaren EA, LeSage B. Feldspathic veneers: what are their indications? Compend Contin Educ Dent 2011;32(3):44–9.
7. Kim J, Chu S, Gurel G, et al. Restorative space management: treatment planning and clinical considerations for insufficient space. Pract Proced Aesthet Dent 2005;17(1):19–25 [quiz: 26].
8. Lowis BR, Gahan MJ, Hodge TM, et al. The orthodontic-restorative interface: 2. Compensating for variations in tooth number and shape. Dent Update 2010; 37(3):138–40, 142-134, 146-138 passim.
9. David SM. Orthodontics & esthetic dentistry: mission possible. J Cosmet Dent 2016;31:14–26.
10. Greenberg JR, Bogert MC. A dental esthetic checklist for treatment planning in esthetic dentistry. Compend Contin Educ Dent 2010;31(8):630–4, 636, 638.
11. Spear FM, Kokich VG, Mathews DP. Interdisciplinary management of anterior dental esthetics. J Am Dent Assoc 2006;137(2):160–9.
12. Brandao RC, Brandao LB. Finishing procedures in orthodontics: dental dimensions and proportions (microesthetics). Dental Press J Orthod 2013;18(5): 147–74.
13. Reikie DF. Orthodontically assisted restorative dentistry. J Can Dent Assoc 2001; 67(9):516–20.
14. Morgano SM, Rodrigues AH, Sabrosa CE. Restoration of endodontically treated teeth. Dent Clin North Am 2004;48(2):vi, 397-416.
15. Kokich V. Esthetics and anterior tooth position: an orthodontic perspective. Part II: Vertical position. J Esthet Dent 1993;5(4):174–8.
16. Salama H, Salama M. The role of orthodontic extrusive remodeling in the enhancement of soft and hard tissue profiles prior to implant placement: a systematic approach to the management of extraction site defects. Int J Periodontics Restorative Dent 1993;13(4):312–33.
17. Borzabadi-Farahani A, Zadeh HH. Adjunctive orthodontic applications in dental implantology. J Oral Implantol 2015;41(4):501–8.
18. Mack MR. Perspective of facial esthetics in dental treatment planning. J Prosthet Dent 1996;75(2):169–76.
19. McLaren EA, Rifkin R. Macroesthetics: facial and dentofacial analysis. J Calif Dent Assoc 2002;30(11):839–46.
20. Rifkin R. Facial analysis: a comprehensive approach to treatment planning in aesthetic dentistry. Pract Periodontics Aesthet Dent 2000;12(9):865–71 [quiz: 872].
21. Coachman C, Calamita M. Digital Smile Design: a tool for treatment planning and communication in esthetic dentistry. QDT 2012;35:103–11.
22. Morley J, Eubank J. Macroesthetic elements of smile design. J Am Dent Assoc 2001;132(1):39–45.
23. Ackerman MB, Ackerman JL. Smile analysis and design in the digital era. J Clin Orthod 2002;36(4):221–36.
24. Proffit WR, Fields HW Jr, et al. Contemporary orthodontics. Elsevier; 2013.
25. Dias NS, Tsingene F. SAEF - Smile's Aesthetic Evaluation Form: a useful tool to improve communication between clinicians and patients during multidisciplinary treatment. Int J Esthet Dent 2011;6(2):160–76.

26. Sarver DM, Ackerman MB. Dynamic smile visualization and quantification: Part 2. Smile analysis and treatment strategies. Am J Orthod Dentofacial Orthop 2003; 124(2):116–27.
27. Sarver DM, Ackerman MB. Dynamic smile visualization and quantification: part 1. Evolution of the concept and dynamic records for smile capture. Am J Orthod Dentofacial Orthop 2003;124(1):4–12.
28. Vig RG, Brundo GC. The kinetics of anterior tooth display. J Prosthet Dent 1978; 39(5):502–4.
29. McLaren EA, Culp L. Smile analysis: the Photoshop smile design. J Cosmet Dent 2013;29:94–108.
30. Lombardi RE. The principles of visual perception and their clinical application to denture esthetics. J Prosthet Dent 1973;29(4):358–82.
31. Davis NC. Smile design. Dent Clin North Am 2007;51(2):299–318, vii.
32. Sarver DM. The importance of incisor positioning in the esthetic smile: the smile arc. Am J Orthod Dentofacial Orthop 2001;120(2):98–111.
33. Magne P, Gallucci GO, Belser UC. Anatomic crown width/length ratios of unworn and worn maxillary teeth in white subjects. J Prosthet Dent 2003;89(5):453–61.
34. Preston JD. The golden proportion revisited. J Esthet Dent 1993;5(6):247–51.
35. Snow SR. Esthetic smile analysis of maxillary anterior tooth width: the golden percentage. J Esthet Dent 1999;11(4):177–84.
36. Ward DH. Proportional smile design using the recurring esthetic dental (red) proportion. Dent Clin North Am 2001;45(1):143–54.
37. Ward DH. A study of dentists' preferred maxillary anterior tooth width proportions: comparing the recurring esthetic dental proportion to other mathematical and naturally occurring proportions. J Esthet Restor Dent 2007;19(6):324–37 [discussion: 338–9].

Branding Dynamics for the Esthetic Dentist

Building Your Brand to Build Your Practice

David J. Wagner, DDS[a,b,*], Julie Logan[c]

KEYWORDS

- Branding • Esthetic dental practice • Professional identity

KEY POINTS

- Branding involves every facet of your professional identity and reputation.
- Powerful and effective branding is a must have in building a thriving esthetic dental practice.
- Powerful and effective branding plays a vital role for patients finding and choosing an esthetic dentist.
- Building your brand requires answering many questions, making many decisions, and implementing those decisions into your personal and professional life.

VALUE OF BRANDING

As dentists, we wear many hats. As clinicians, we perform a variety of procedures we learn in dental school, advanced training programs, and continuing education courses. As practice owners, whether in solo or partnered practices, there is another set of critical skills for which we have little to no training.

When operating in the esthetic dental arena, there is a shift in the way that patients find a provider. Esthetic dentistry is like any other elective or luxury purchase: perception and emotion play a key role in consumer decision-making and patronage. When looking for a dentist who is excellent at elective procedures that involve improving appearance, patients look for a dentist who not only has a sound reputation and experience, but also one who has an elevated visual presence online, and elsewhere, representing their skills, work, esthetic style, and practice environment.

---

[a] Private Practice, West Hollywood, CA, USA; [b] UCLA Center for Esthetic Dentistry; [c] Writing and Branding Consultant based in Los Angeles, USA
* Corresponding author. 8733 Beverly Boulevard #202, West Hollywood, CA 90048.
E-mail address: drwagner@pinarwagner.com

Dent Clin N Am 64 (2020) 731–737
https://doi.org/10.1016/j.cden.2020.07.001
0011-8532/20/© 2020 Elsevier Inc. All rights reserved.

dental.theclinics.com

After years of education and training, it can be surprising and frustrating to young dentists looking to add an esthetic component to their practice that their skills may not be the metric by which prospective patients choose to call their office, seek their services, or schedule a procedure. The reality is that few people outside the dental field can truly understand the many factors that define clinical excellence and optimal natural-looking esthetic treatment. The metric that patients must go by is purely our reputation based on a referral or the image created by branding and marketing efforts that emotionally communicates our skills, our style, and our commitment to caring, ethical, and outstanding treatment outcomes.

A promotional piece from the Digital Smile Design Company speaks to this point:

> As dentists we invest time and money honing our clinical skills. However, when it comes to making a decision about a treatment plan, patients don't consider your advanced skill in occlusion, nor your training in teeth preparation. In fact, whenever a patient makes a decision about treatment, it's always a leap of faith – even if you have 100 diplomas on your clinic wall.[1]

EMOTIONAL CONNECTION

To attract prospective patients to your practice and motivate them to accept treatment with you, these patients have to *believe* you can deliver the results they desire. For them to stay motivated and compliant throughout treatment involving irreversible changes to their appearance, significant out-of-pocket investment, and multiple visits over a period of time, they have to *trust* you and the process. To foster that belief and trust from others, you have to portray an imagine of yourself as highly competent, likable, and ethical: a true expert. This means that determining and defining who and what you are, branding, is as equally important as honing clinical skills to be a successful esthetic dentist.

Done well, branding also sets you apart from your competition, as it emphasizes your superior points of difference. Once you are clear about your brand, it becomes not only easier for you to communicate who you are and what you do, but for others (patients, colleagues, media, family, and friends) to understand you and your practice and therefore choose you over others.

Although many branded components (printed pieces, social media, signage, and promotion) involve language, ultimately what branding does is communicate in ways that go deeper than language. Its currency is feeling and impression. When you are on target, belief, trust, and connection follow naturally for both existing and prospective patients as well as for your colleagues and community. Like attracts like, and therefore if your branding is sophisticated, elegant, and warm, you are going to attract a patient base that responds to businesses and messaging that are sophisticated, elegant, and warm.

BRANDING DEFINITION

'Branding' is one of those terms so overused it has almost become meaningless and can be confusing. Also confusing to the uninitiated is that branding has its own vocabulary (See Appendix 1). The actual meaning fundamentally can be looked at in two ways.

Short definition: *Branding defines identity*.

Longer definition: *Branding expresses identity via goods, services, environments, and behaviors (and often a combination of the 4) across multiple platforms and in multiple contexts*. In other words, branding works to create a single identity encapsulating every single thing a dentist and dental practice would say, be, do, offer, display, look like, occupy, or make.

There are certain characteristics and qualities that define branding. Good branding is the *consistent* or *logical* identity expression across every platform and context that is executed with simplicity and clarity. Every element syncs with or makes perfect sense with the other. This means that your services, your logo design, your social media, your practice's décor, printed patient aftercare information, your staff scrubs, and your promotional videos line up with each other to consistently portray your personality and message. These are all examples of physical branding components.

It is critical to understand that branding for dentists transcends the tangible, where it also heavily involves your personal and professional reputation. In addition, it involves every interaction a patient has with your practice, including the moment any team member starts interacting with a prospective or current patient: online, on the phone, or in person. The less friction a patient encounters to learn about your identity, find your practice location, and schedule an appointment, the better; the level of friction is reflective of your brand. Both tangible and intangible aspects of brand will help reduce points of friction for patients, giving them a better experience. A clearly written web site explains your services, whereas your front office team clearly explaining the consultation process and value of your high-level services are both integral to instill enough emotional excitement in a patient leading them to choose you.

Brian Collins, founder of the eponymous Collins, a "strategy and brand-experience design company based in San Francisco, who works with some of the world's best brands including Spotify, Nike, and The San Francisco Symphony," says this about brand: "From the moment that you start talking about your company, launch a web site or have someone answer your phone, there's a brand there. So my argument is simple: be conscious of it. Protect it. Manage it like you would any valuable asset."[2]

Branding a dental practice is similar to other industries in that the physical and visual presence is critical. However, it is also unique in that we are health care professionals, and our reputation as compassionate, caring, and ethical individuals when interacting with patients, as well as in our professional and local communities matters equally. Successful dentists fully understand that both facets, the physical and interpersonal, are critical to their brand building and will constantly work to develop not only their own skills but also the skills of their entire team and practice culture.

BEGINNING THE BRANDING JOURNEY

Powerful branding begins with astute analysis of self and goals. Developing a brand requires a detailed, organized strategy and a tremendous amount of focus and preparation. The amount of detail and effort that goes into developing a good brand is often underappreciated and undervalued, mainly due to a lack of understanding by people outside of the branding field. This is where we as esthetic dentists are at a distinct advantage. One thing we do particularly well is focus, deriving precise information (esthetically, technically, practically, and even emotionally) from what we observe and subsequently conclude. As a dentist, creating your brand can be done in several ways: done by yourself, by enlisting the services of a branding professional or agency, or some combination of the two. Regardless of your desired investment, there is a general, logical sequence that is pursued to have a brand be realized. Each step of the process gets you closer and closer to your end goal of an overall cohesive and recognizable identity.

Typically when starting the branding journey, a document called a *brand brief* is used as a beginning point. A brand brief contains a number of questions that must be answered to start to formulate exactly who you are, inform your vision, map out how you want to be perceived, and define the demographics of your desired prospective patients so they can be targeted with your marketing and media efforts. Without the brand brief as a foundation, efforts to attract and impress patients become disjointed and unclear, leading to confusion and potential clients moving on. Just like a great film starts with a powerful script, so does a great brand begin with a powerful brand brief.

HIRING PROFESSIONALS

Implementing a good branding program does take a considerable amount of work. It is a commitment requiring a significant amount of time, money, and concentration. It may also mean securing the talents of a branding professional, graphic designer, web site designer, social media specialist, interior designer, and perhaps even an advertising agency, marketing specialist, videographer, or copywriter.

You do not necessarily need to find each of these on your own, although you may choose a do-it-yourself (DIY) approach is perfectly acceptable and can reduce investment. However, a DIY approach will require much more time, organization, and research on the dentist's part to properly execute a cohesive brand. If you hire a branding company, agency, or studio, it will take on the role of project manager to find and coordinate many of the various creative elements. Some companies offer a comprehensive, templated one-size-fits-all package. This may work for this with less time or money. However, just like in esthetic dentistry and other elective goods and services, the higher the sensibility and sophistication, the more investment required.

A reliable metric for hiring compatible creative professionals is to determine if they are as good at what they do as you are what you do. Looking at specific examples of a branding expert's previous work will help determine if their style and esthetic aligns with your vision. Although each branding project done by a professional should be unique and individualized, the overall skill level and ability of the branding professional to sculpt an identity for themselves can be assessed and is also something on which to base a decision.

The other group of individuals that must be involved when executing high-level branding is your team, because they are, in fact, the most important part of your brand. Developing your practice's branding is not something you want to do in isolation and then spring on your team after the fact. From the outset, you need every single member of your team to participate, understand, value, support, and perhaps even help build your practice's vision and mission. Branding should be a topic of discussion at every team meeting, along with public acknowledgment of those with good ideas.

As time goes on, a brand becomes a living, breathing, evolving entity and must be managed by those individuals involved in the day-to-day operations of the practice. This evolution happens as services are added, systems improve, clientele demographics shift, and ultimately the practice elevates its status. Involving the team from the outset results in them taking a significant interest, understanding, and ownership of the brand and therefore a vested interest in the growth and overall well-being of the practice. Team members can be encouraged to fill out the brand development worksheets shown later in this article.

An important point to make is that you may already employ individuals who have a talent for branding ideas and analysis. Sometimes an astute team member will know you better than you know yourself and offer valuable insights. A team member who has an affinity for photography and social media, for example, can best put those interests to work to regularly manage your practice's content while you are busy seeing patients and producing.

RETURN ON INVESTMENT

In developing a personal strategy to complete a new or re-brand of your practice, budgets are of primary concern. One of the worksheets found later in this article, which will take a fair amount of research and at least a few weeks to complete, will help you work to find the creative and technical professionals (and style) you like and the costs for each service. Learning all this at the outset will prevent financial surprises later and allow you to plan. It is not uncommon to break up the branding process into affordable pieces. From there, you will be able to determine who is worth what to you and your practice. It is also important to note that all possible aspects of branding do not need to be executed for all dental practices. For example, an esthetic dental practice may find significant value in social media video content in ways that other practices or specialists may not. Once you have developed your brand, market research continues the process to effectively put the brand to work.

SUMMARY

As you start to think about your brand, a strategic mix of the personal, the professional, and the practice, remind yourself that you are unique, complete with a specific combination of skills, experience, and personality. You have come so far but there is still work to do. Authentically branding yourself now will be the next step on the road to greater success.

DISCLOSURE

The authors have nothing to disclose.

REFERENCES

1. Digital Smile Design. What is an emotional presentation and how can it change the way your patients connect with you?. Available at: https://media. digitalsmiledesign.com/news/what-is-an-emotional-presentation. Accessed April 23, 2020.

2. Collins B. How to find your brand. Monocle 2020;19.

APPENDIX 1:

Branding Glossary

When you first meet with branding professionals, and these can include agencies, social media consultants, copywriters, graphic designers, and videographers, they are likely to use terminology that is unfamiliar to you. Here are a few insider terms to get you started:

Brand: an entity's identity incorporating a mix of tangible and intangible attributes. Although it is most often the physical representation of a company's esthetic, offerings, and values, it can also exist subjectively in a person's mind.

Branding: the act of creating, selecting, and blending attributes to differentiate a product, service, or business.

Good branding: consistency of image and identity across various platforms in an attractive, meaningful, and compelling way to attract and build loyalty with a specific, targeted customer base.

Brand brief: a document that spells out all the attributes a company wants articulated by their branding.

Brand book: also known as a style guide or brand bible, a document that illustrates all philosophic and visual aspects of a brand, including identity and values statements, target

market information, graphic design, proper logo application, templates, color palette, typography, and media.
Collateral: digital and printed pieces, such as brochures, post cards, and signage.
CTA: call to action. All digital media and collateral pieces should feature a CTA, that is, a clear indication of what they want the reader/viewer to do (as in sign up, call, schedule, purchase, order, or respond.)
Mission statement: defines the present state or purpose of a company, service, or product. It answers three essential questions: WHAT it does; WHO it does it for; and HOW it does what it does. Written succinctly in the form of a sentence or two, the mission statement is something that all employees should be able to recite on request.
Vision statement: inward-facing company-eyes-only articulation of desired outcome over time, its metric for success. These goals can be abstract or tied to something specific, like customer base or a dollar figure.
Core values statement: a list of a company's non-negotiable characteristics regarding ethical business practices, quality delivery, customer service, diversity, sustainability, transparency, staff support, and kindness.

BRANDING DOs AND DONTs

- DO remember that branding is a work in progress, you might not get it exactly right the first time and your brand may change over time.
- DON'T try to do all of your branding at once especially if you don't have the time or the budget.
- DO approach your brand developing every day, even if it is only in 30-minute or even 15-minute increments at a time. In fact, good ideas often come to you between sessions but only if you keep them up frequently enough to build momentum.
- DO always move forward with analysis and writing down your answers step by step.
- DO learn to articulate *why* you like something or do not like something. Although it may not come naturally in the beginning, you will get better at this as you go along.
- DO interview and comparison shop multiple candidates/companies for any professional service you hire
- DO help the decision-making process by finding multiple examples (even outside the dentistry field) that reflect your taste and goals and compare them with each other. Show these examples to any professionals you are interviewing or have hired to help you. Good examples may be specific brands you love, such as a technology, clothing, shoes, or automobile media content, such as their social media posts or in print campaigns.

WORK SHEETS

Brand development means asking questions, answering them, and then basing your plans of action on what you have learned. The good news is that thinking, planning, and envisioning are free. The more you have figured out in advance, the more astute you will be in controlling the narrative moving forward. Always remember the most effective communication is simple and direct.

Preliminary Exploration: What Does Your Profile Look Like?
The descriptive words you note below can be real or aspirational. These can range from technical to aesthetic to emotional. Feel free to revise this list or add other categories as you go along. For added insight, you can also ask members of your staff to complete this exercise too.

For *each* of the following, note *five adjectives* that describe
- You personally
- You professionally
- Your practice's technology and equipment
- Your practice culture
- Your office's décor and environment
- Your practice's communication materials, both printed and digital
- Your colleagues
- Your staff
- Your team training
- Your traditional media and promotion
- Your social media and digital communication

Conclusion: By compiling these you will be building your practice branding profile. Certain themes will emerge. This profile will function as your branding benchmark by which you judge every decision you make. Does it sync, does it go, does it work, does it make sense?

Components, Professional Wish List, and Budget
For each of the following, find at least three examples of other brands you like and three you do not like. Make a spreadsheet on which you note the following:
a. What you like or do not like and *specifically* why.
b. On the ones you like, find out who created them and their contact details.
c. On the ones you like, note the cost. You may be unable to find this information.
d. Because you are breaking out each and every one of these items individually (and doing it three times per), do not be surprised at the heft of the document.

This can also serve as a checklist for areas of branding. You may not need all of these. You may have additional components you desire.

Some of these (advertising, for example) have multiple parts requiring individual pricing.

2-Dimensional design
__ GRAPHIC DESIGN (logo, business cards, letterhead, printed and digital materials including social media formatted posts)
__ INTAKE FORMS (digital or printed)
__ BROCHURES AND POSTCARDS
__ PATIENT FOLDER AND FORMS
__ ADVERTISING (if yes, where, with whom and what are your desired results?)
__ COPYWRITING (optional, if no, who is going to do it?)

Media and social media
__ WEB SITE DESIGN
__ MONTHLY WEBMASTER MAINTENANCE
__ PHOTOGRAPHY
__ VIDEOGRAPHY
__ MONTHLY SOCIAL MEDIA MANAGEMENT
__ MONTHLY PUBLIC RELATIONS (if yes, where, with whom and what are your desired results?)

Dress, décor, and atmosphere
__ INTERIOR DESIGN
__ SCRUBS, UNIFORMS, AND DRESS CODE
__ MUSIC
__ MEDIA (video)

Staff training and education
__ STAFF SCRIPTS
__ OUTSIDE PRESENTATIONS

UNITED STATES POSTAL SERVICE ®

Statement of Ownership, Management, and Circulation
(All Periodicals Publications Except Requester Publications)

1. Publication Title	2. Publication Number		3. Filing Date
DENTAL CLINICS OF NORTH AMERICA	566 – 480		9/18/2020

4. Issue Frequency	5. Number of Issues Published Annually	6. Annual Subscription Price
JAN, APR, JUL, OCT	4	$304.00

7. Complete Mailing Address of Known Office of Publication (Not printer) (Street, city, county, state, and ZIP+4®)

ELSEVIER INC.
230 Park Avenue, Suite 800
New York, NY 10169

Contact Person
Malathi Samayan

Telephone (Include area code)
91-44-4299-4507

8. Complete Mailing Address of Headquarters or General Business Office of Publisher (Not printer)

ELSEVIER INC.
230 Park Avenue, Suite 800
New York, NY 10169

9. Full Names and Complete Mailing Addresses of Publisher, Editor, and Managing Editor (Do not leave blank)

Publisher (Name and complete mailing address)

DOLORES MELONI, ELSEVIER INC.
1600 JOHN F KENNEDY BLVD. SUITE 1800
PHILADELPHIA, PA 19103-2899

Editor (Name and complete mailing address)

JOHN VASSALLO, ELSEVIER INC.
1600 JOHN F KENNEDY BLVD. SUITE 1800
PHILADELPHIA, PA 19103-2899

Managing Editor (Name and complete mailing address)

PATRICK MANLEY, ELSEVIER INC.
1600 JOHN F KENNEDY BLVD. SUITE 1800
PHILADELPHIA, PA 19103-2899

10. Owner (Do not leave blank. If the publication is owned by a corporation, give the name and address of the corporation immediately followed by the names and addresses of all stockholders owning or holding 1 percent or more of the total amount of stock. If not owned by a corporation, give the names and addresses of the individual owners. If owned by a partnership or other unincorporated firm, give its name and address as well as those of each individual owner. If the publication is published by a nonprofit organization, give its name and address.)

Full Name	Complete Mailing Address
WHOLLY OWNED SUBSIDIARY OF REED/ELSEVIER, US HOLDINGS	1600 JOHN F KENNEDY BLVD. SUITE 1800 PHILADELPHIA, PA 19103-2899

11. Known Bondholders, Mortgagees, and Other Security Holders Owning or Holding 1 Percent or More of Total Amount of Bonds, Mortgages, or Other Securities. If none, check box → ☐ None

Full Name	Complete Mailing Address
N/A	

12. Tax Status (For completion by nonprofit organizations authorized to mail at nonprofit rates) (Check one)
The purpose, function, and nonprofit status of this organization and the exempt status for federal income tax purposes:
☒ Has Not Changed During Preceding 12 Months
☐ Has Changed During Preceding 12 Months (Publisher must submit explanation of change with this statement)

PS Form **3526**, July 2014 [Page 1 of 4 (see instructions page 4)] PSN: 7530-01-000-9931 PRIVACY NOTICE: See our privacy policy on www.usps.com

13. Publication Title	14. Issue Date for Circulation Data Below
DENTAL CLINICS OF NORTH AMERICA	JULY 2020

15. Extent and Nature of Circulation		Average No. Copies Each Issue During Preceding 12 Months	No. Copies of Single Issue Published Nearest to Filing Date
a. Total Number of Copies (Net press run)		247	210
b. Paid Circulation (By Mail and Outside the Mail)	(1) Mailed Outside-County Paid Subscriptions Stated on PS Form 3541 (include paid distribution above nominal rate, advertiser's proof copies, and exchange copies)	137	121
	(2) Mailed In-County Paid Subscriptions Stated on PS Form 3541 (include paid distribution above nominal rate, advertiser's proof copies, and exchange copies)	0	0
	(3) Paid Distribution Outside the Mails Including Sales Through Dealers and Carriers, Street Vendors, Counter Sales, and Other Paid Distribution Outside USPS®	77	52
	(4) Paid Distribution by Other Classes of Mail Through the USPS (e.g. First-Class Mail®)	0	0
c. Total Paid Distribution (Sum of 15b (1), (2), (3), and (4))	▶	214	173
d. Free or Nominal Rate Distribution (By Mail and Outside the Mail)	(1) Free or Nominal Rate Outside-County Copies included on PS Form 3541	18	20
	(2) Free or Nominal Rate In-County Copies Included on PS Form 3541	0	0
	(3) Free or Nominal Rate Copies Mailed at Other Classes Through the USPS (e.g. First-Class Mail)	0	0
	(4) Free or Nominal Rate Distribution Outside the Mail (Carriers or other means)	0	0
e. Total Free or Nominal Rate Distribution (Sum of 15d (1), (2), (3) and (4))	▶	18	20
f. Total Distribution (Sum of 15c and 15e)	▶	232	193
g. Copies not Distributed (See Instructions to Publishers #4 (page #3))	▶	15	17
h. Total (Sum of 15f and g)	▶	247	210
i. Percent Paid (15c divided by 15f times 100)		92.24%	89.63%

* If you are claiming electronic copies, go to line 16 on page 3. If you are not claiming electronic copies, skip to line 17 on page 3.

16. Electronic Copy Circulation		Average No. Copies Each Issue During Preceding 12 Months	No. Copies of Single Issue Published Nearest to Filing Date
a. Paid Electronic Copies	▶		
b. Total Paid Print Copies (Line 15c) + Paid Electronic Copies (Line 16a)	▶		
c. Total Print Distribution (Line 15f) + Paid Electronic Copies (Line 16a)	▶		
d. Percent Paid (Both Print & Electronic Copies) (16b divided by 16c × 100)	▶		

☒ I certify that 50% of all my distributed copies (electronic and print) are paid above a nominal price.

17. Publication of Statement of Ownership

☒ If the publication is a general publication, publication of this statement is required. Will be printed in the OCTOBER 2020 issue of this publication.
☐ Publication not required.

18. Signature and Title of Editor, Publisher, Business Manager, or Owner	Date
Malathi Samayan - Distribution Controller	*Malathi Samayan*	9/18/2020

I certify that all information furnished on this form is true and complete. I understand that anyone who furnishes false or misleading information on this form or who omits material or information requested on the form may be subject to criminal sanctions (including fines and imprisonment) and/or civil sanctions (including civil penalties).

PS Form **3526**, July 2014 (Page 3 of 4) PRIVACY NOTICE: See our privacy policy on www.usps.com

Printed and bound by CPI Group (UK) Ltd, Croydon, CR0 4YY

03/10/2024

01040479-0012